C000008040

UK Ambulance Services
Clinical Practice
Guidelines 2013

POCKET BOOK

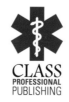

CLASS
PROFESSIONAL
PUBLISHING

Disclaimer

This Pocket Book has been produced by AACE and JRCALC and is based on the UK Ambulance Services Clinical Practice Guidelines 2013 (Reference Edition) v1.1. This is the second print run and contains some minor amendments and adjustments to the layout within the page for age section. The Pocket Book is intended to be used by clinicians working in the prehospital setting to confirm safe therapeutic drug dosages prior to administration. It also contains treatment algorithms and management plans that are intended to be used as a quick reference guide only. As such it is designed to be used in conjunction with the Reference Edition of the UK Ambulance Services Clinical Practice Guidelines 2013 which contain the definitive text that cannot be reproduced in this Pocket Book.

The Association of Ambulance Chief Executives and the Joint Royal Colleges Ambulance Liaison Committee have made every effort to ensure that the information, tables, drawings and diagrams contained in these guidelines are accurate at the time of publication. However, the 2013 guidelines are advisory and have been developed to assist healthcare professionals, and patients, to make decisions about the management of the patient's health, including treatments. This advice is intended to support the decision making process and is not a substitute for sound clinical judgement. The guidelines cannot always contain all the information necessary for determining appropriate care and cannot address all individual situations; therefore, individuals using these guidelines must ensure they have the appropriate knowledge and skills to enable suitable interpretation.

The Association of Ambulance Chief Executives does not guarantee, and accepts no legal liability of whatever nature arising from or connected to, the accuracy, reliability, currency or completeness of the content of these guidelines.

Users of these guidelines must always be aware that such innovations or alterations after the date of publication may not be incorporated in the content. As part of its commitment to defining national standards, the association will periodically issue updates to the content and users should ensure that they are using the most up-to-date version of the guidelines. These updates can be found on www.aaceguidelines.co.uk. Please note however that the Association of Ambulance Chief Executives assumes no responsibility whatsoever for the content of external resources.

Although some modification of the guidelines may be required by individual ambulance services, and approved by the relevant local clinical committees, to ensure they respond to the health requirements of the local community, the majority of the guidance is universally applicable to NHS ambulance services. Modification of the guidelines may also occur when undertaking research sanctioned by a research ethics committee.

Whilst these guidelines cover the full range of paramedic treatments available across the UK they will also provide a valuable tool for ambulance technicians and other prehospital providers. Many of the assessment skills and general principles will remain the same. Those not qualified to paramedic level must practise within their level of training and competence.

The information presented in this book is accurate and current to the best of the authors' knowledge. The authors and publisher, however, make no guarantee as to, and assume no responsibility for, the correctness, sufficiency or completeness of such information or recommendation.

Printing history
First edition published 2013, reprinted 2013, 2015 (Version 1.2).
The content for Reference Edition 1.3 and Pocket Book 1.2 was updated in January 2015.

The authors and publisher welcome feedback from the users of this book.
Please contact the publisher:
Class Professional Publishing,
The Exchange, Express Park, Bristol Road, Bridgwater TA6 4RR
Telephone: 01278 427843   Email: post@class.co.uk
Website: www.classprofessional.co.uk

Class Professional Publishing is an imprint of Class Publishing Ltd

A CIP catalogue record for this book is available from the British Library
ISBN 978 185959 365 3

Designed and typeset by Typematter

Project managed by Cambridge Publishing Management Limited

Line illustrations by David Woodroffe

Printed and bound in Italy by L.E.G.O.

This edition:
UK Ambulance Services Clinical Practice Guidelines 2013 Pocket Book
ISBN 978 185959 365 3 (print edition)

Also available:
UK Ambulance Services Clinical Practice Guidelines 2013 Pocket Book
ISBN 978 185959 366 0 (e-book)

UK Ambulance Services Clinical Practice Guidelines 2013 Reference Edition
ISBN 978 185959 363 9 (print edition)

UK Ambulance Services Clinical Practice Guidelines 2013 Reference Edition
ISBN 978 185959 364 6 (e-book)

For free updates, and details of how to order, go to: www.AACEGuidelines.co.uk

RESUSCITATION

Basic Life Support (Adult)

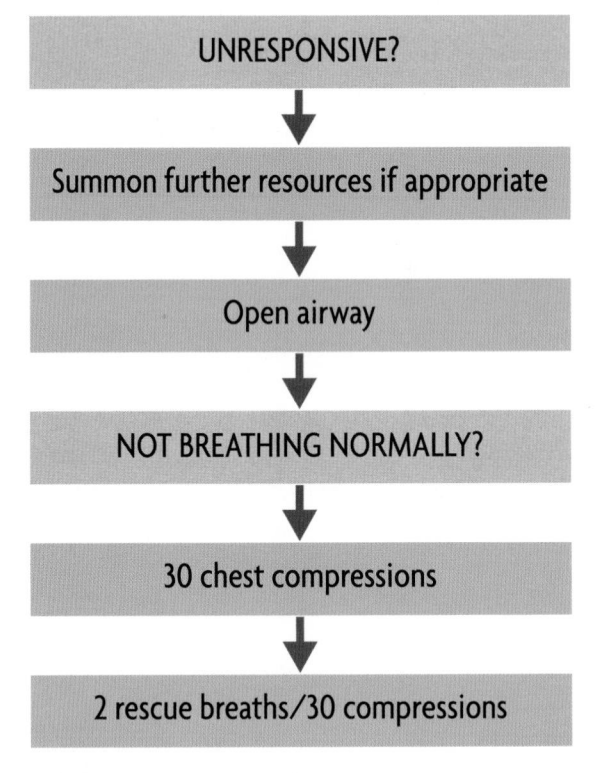

Advanced Life Support (Adult)

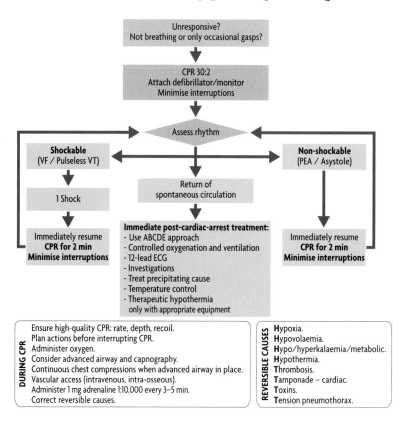

Unresponsive?
Not breathing or only occasional gasps?

↓

CPR 30:2
Attach defibrillator/monitor
Minimise interruptions

↓

Assess rhythm

Shockable
(VF / Pulseless VT)

↓

1 Shock

↓

Immediately resume
**CPR for 2 min
Minimise interruptions**

Return of
spontaneous circulation

Immediate post-cardiac-arrest treatment:
- Use ABCDE approach
- Controlled oxygenation and ventilation
- 12-lead ECG
- Investigations
- Treat precipitating cause
- Temperature control
- Therapeutic hypothermia
  only with appropriate equipment

Non-shockable
(PEA / Asystole)

↓

Immediately resume
**CPR for 2 min
Minimise interruptions**

DURING CPR

Ensure high-quality CPR: rate, depth, recoil.
Plan actions before interrupting CPR.
Administer oxygen.
Consider advanced airway and capnography.
Continuous chest compressions when advanced airway in place.
Vascular access (intravenous, intra-osseous).
Administer 1 mg adrenaline 1:10,000 every 3–5 min.
Correct reversible causes.

REVERSIBLE CAUSES

Hypoxia.
Hypovolaemia.
Hypo/hyperkalaemia/metabolic.
Hypothermia.
Thrombosis.
Tamponade – cardiac.
Toxins.
Tension pneumothorax.

Airway and Breathing Management

Airway assessment and management overview.

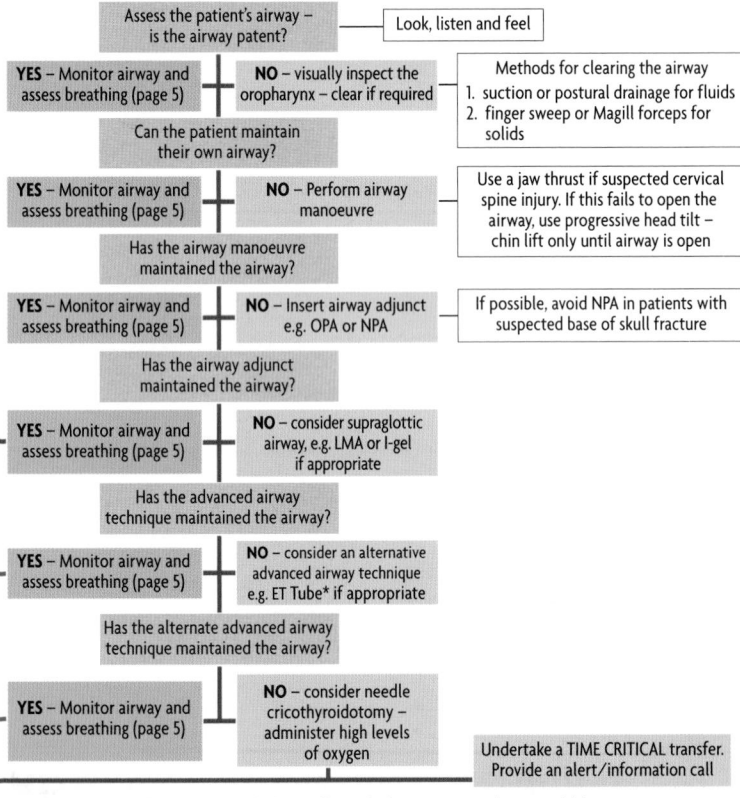

Assess the patient's airway – is the airway patent? —— Look, listen and feel

YES – Monitor airway and assess breathing (page 5) —— **NO** – visually inspect the oropharynx – clear if required

Methods for clearing the airway
1. suction or postural drainage for fluids
2. finger sweep or Magill forceps for solids

Can the patient maintain their own airway?

YES – Monitor airway and assess breathing (page 5) —— **NO** – Perform airway manoeuvre

Use a jaw thrust if suspected cervical spine injury. If this fails to open the airway, use progressive head tilt – chin lift only until airway is open

Has the airway manoeuvre maintained the airway?

YES – Monitor airway and assess breathing (page 5) —— **NO** – Insert airway adjunct e.g. OPA or NPA

If possible, avoid NPA in patients with suspected base of skull fracture

Has the airway adjunct maintained the airway?

YES – Monitor airway and assess breathing (page 5) —— **NO** – consider supraglottic airway, e.g. LMA or I-gel if appropriate

Has the advanced airway technique maintained the airway?

YES – Monitor airway and assess breathing (page 5) —— **NO** – consider an alternative advanced airway technique e.g. ET Tube* if appropriate

Has the alternate advanced airway technique maintained the airway?

YES – Monitor airway and assess breathing (page 5) —— **NO** – consider needle cricothyroidotomy – administer high levels of oxygen

Undertake a TIME CRITICAL transfer. Provide an alert/information call

*Endotracheal intubation must only be performed when capnography is available.

Airway and Breathing Management

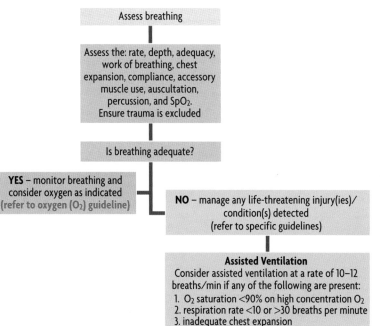

Assess breathing

Assess the: rate, depth, adequacy, work of breathing, chest expansion, compliance, accessory muscle use, auscultation, percussion, and SpO₂. Ensure trauma is excluded

Is breathing adequate?

YES – monitor breathing and consider oxygen as indicated (refer to oxygen (O₂) guideline)

NO – manage any life-threatening injury(ies)/condition(s) detected (refer to specific guidelines)

Assisted Ventilation
Consider assisted ventilation at a rate of 10–12 breaths/min if any of the following are present:
1. O₂ saturation <90% on high concentration O₂
2. respiration rate <10 or >30 breaths per minute
3. inadequate chest expansion

If the patient has life-threatening injury(ies)/condition(s) or is receiving ventilatory assistance undertake a TIME CRITICAL transfer. Provide an alert/information call

Recognition of Life Extinct by Ambulance Clinicians

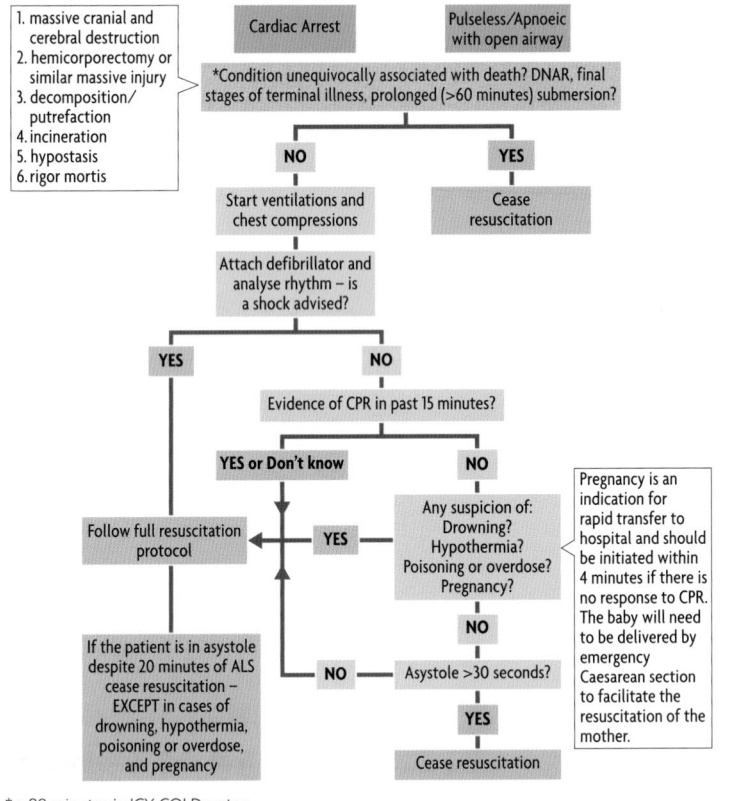

1. massive cranial and cerebral destruction
2. hemicorporectomy or similar massive injury
3. decomposition/putrefaction
4. incineration
5. hypostasis
6. rigor mortis

Cardiac Arrest

Pulseless/Apnoeic with open airway

*Condition unequivocally associated with death? DNAR, final stages of terminal illness, prolonged (>60 minutes) submersion?

NO

YES

Start ventilations and chest compressions

Cease resuscitation

Attach defibrillator and analyse rhythm – is a shock advised?

YES

NO

Evidence of CPR in past 15 minutes?

YES or Don't know

NO

Follow full resuscitation protocol

Any suspicion of:
Drowning?
Hypothermia?
Poisoning or overdose?
Pregnancy?

YES

NO

If the patient is in asystole despite 20 minutes of ALS cease resuscitation – EXCEPT in cases of drowning, hypothermia, poisoning or overdose, and pregnancy

NO

Asystole >30 seconds?

YES

Cease resuscitation

Pregnancy is an indication for rapid transfer to hospital and should be initiated within 4 minutes if there is no response to CPR. The baby will need to be delivered by emergency Caesarean section to facilitate the resuscitation of the mother.

* >90 minutes in ICY COLD water.

Action to be Taken after Verification of Fact of Death

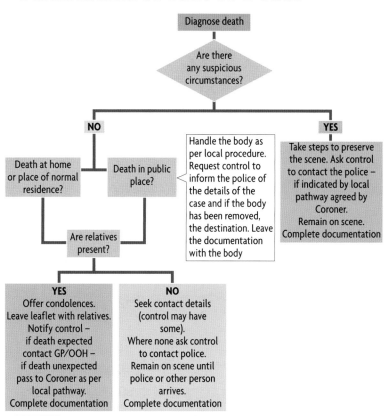

Diagnose death

Are there any suspicious circumstances?

NO

Death at home or place of normal residence?

Death in public place?

Handle the body as per local procedure. Request control to inform the police of the details of the case and if the body has been removed, the destination. Leave the documentation with the body

YES

Take steps to preserve the scene. Ask control to contact the police – if indicated by local pathway agreed by Coroner. Remain on scene. Complete documentation

Are relatives present?

YES
Offer condolences. Leave leaflet with relatives. Notify control – if death expected contact GP/OOH – if death unexpected pass to Coroner as per local pathway. Complete documentation

NO
Seek contact details (control may have some). Where none ask control to contact police. Remain on scene until police or other person arrives. Complete documentation

The Implantable Cardioverter Defibrillator

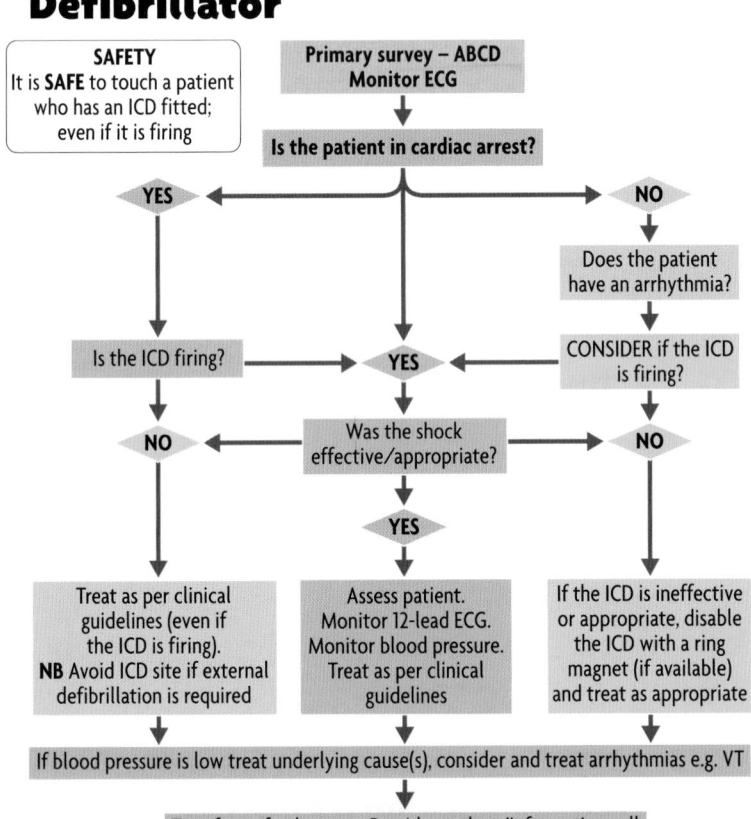

SAFETY
It is **SAFE** to touch a patient who has an ICD fitted; even if it is firing

Primary survey – ABCD Monitor ECG

Is the patient in cardiac arrest?

YES

NO

Does the patient have an arrhythmia?

Is the ICD firing?

YES

CONSIDER if the ICD is firing?

NO

Was the shock effective/appropriate?

NO

YES

Treat as per clinical guidelines (even if the ICD is firing).
NB Avoid ICD site if external defibrillation is required

Assess patient. Monitor 12-lead ECG. Monitor blood pressure. Treat as per clinical guidelines

If the ICD is ineffective or appropriate, disable the ICD with a ring magnet (if available) and treat as appropriate

If blood pressure is low treat underlying cause(s), consider and treat arrhythmias e.g. VT

Transfer to further care. Provide an alert/information call

Foreign Body Airway Obstruction (Adult)

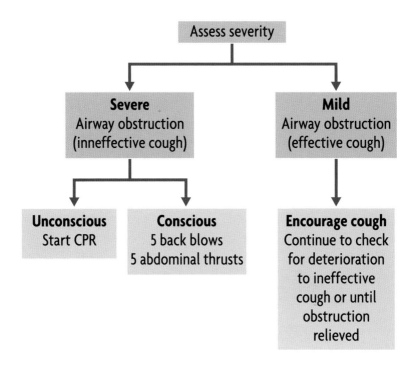

GENERAL

Pain Management in Adults

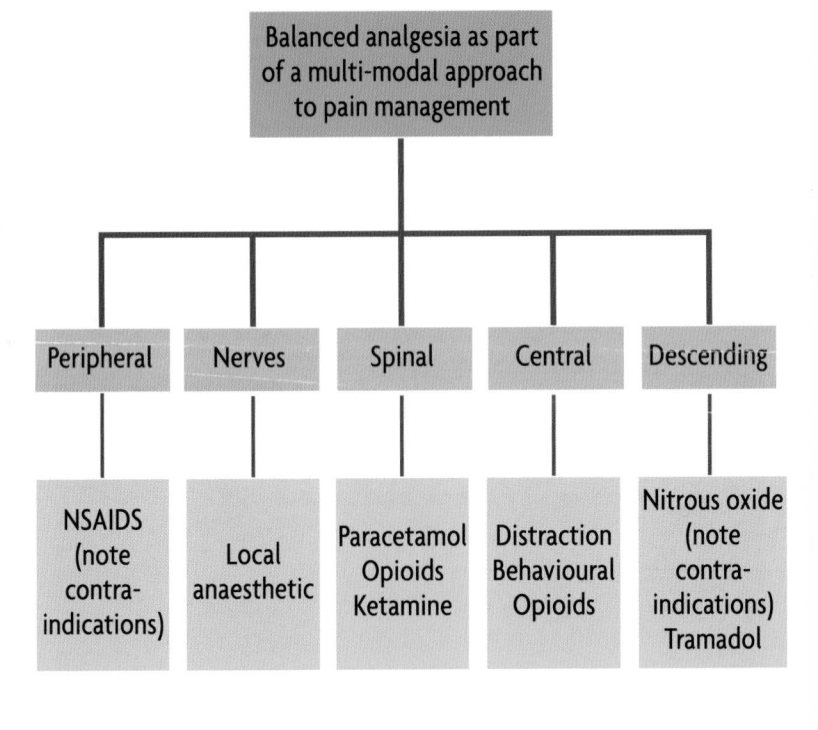

Pain Assessment Model

S	Site	Where exactly is the pain?
O	Onset	What were they doing when the pain started?
C	Character	What does the pain feel like?
R	Radiates	Does the pain go anywhere else?
A	Associated symptoms	e.g. nausea/vomiting
T	Time/duration	How long have they had the pain?
E	Exacerbating/ relieving factors	Does anything make the pain better or worse?
S	Severity	Obtain an initial pain score

Glasgow Coma Scale

Category	Element	Score
Eyes Opening	Spontaneously	4
	To speech	3
	To pain	2
	None	1
Motor Response	Obeys commands	6
	Localises pain	5
	Withdraws from pain	4
	Abnormal flexion	3
	Extensor response	2
	No response to pain	1
Verbal Response	Orientated	5
	Confused	4
	Inappropriate words	3
	Incomprehensible sounds	2
	No verbal response	1

Suicide and Self-Harm Risk Assessment Form

Item	Value	Patient Score
Sex: female	0	
Sex: male	1	
Age: less than 19 years old	1	
Age: greater than 45 years old	1	
Depression/hopelessness	1	
Previous attempts at self-harm	1	
Evidence of excess alcohol/illicit drug use	1	
Rational thinking absent	1	
Separated/divorced/widowed	1	
Organised or serious self-harm	1	
No close/reliable family, job or active religious affiliation	1	
Determined to repeat or ambivalent	1	

Total score of patient

< 3 = Low Risk,   3–6 = Medium Risk,   > 6 = High Risk

MEDICAL

Acute Coronary Syndrome

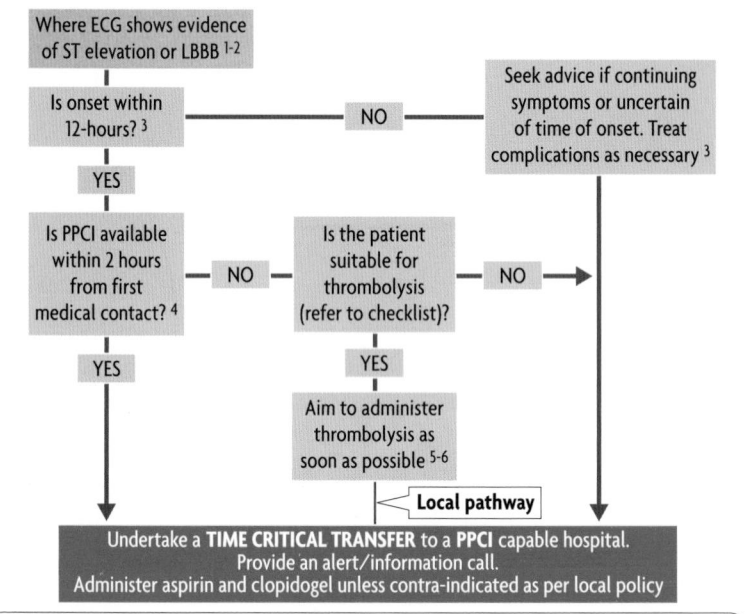

Where ECG shows evidence of ST elevation or LBBB [1-2]

Is onset within 12-hours? [3] — **NO** → Seek advice if continuing symptoms or uncertain of time of onset. Treat complications as necessary [3]

YES

Is PPCI available within 2 hours from first medical contact? [4] — **NO** → Is the patient suitable for thrombolysis (refer to checklist)? — **NO** →

YES

YES (under thrombolysis question) → Aim to administer thrombolysis as soon as possible [5-6]

Local pathway

Undertake a **TIME CRITICAL TRANSFER** to a **PPCI** capable hospital.
Provide an alert/information call.
Administer aspirin and clopidogel unless contra-indicated as per local policy

---

1. Up to a third of patients with MI will have atypical presentations such as shortness of breath or collapse, without chest pain. This is particularly so in patients with diabetes or the elderly. **Have a low threshold for performing a 12-lead ECG in any patient presenting as 'unwell'.** Seek advice in 'atypical' patients who have ST elevation or LBBB (see below) as urgent reperfusion may still be indicated.

2. ECG criteria for reperfusion include ST segment elevation (≥ 2 mm in 2-standard or 2 adjacent precordial leads, not including V1) or **LBBB** in patients with other clinical features suggestive of ACS. Patients who have ST depression rather than elevation are a high risk group who need urgent specialist assessment. **Seek advice.**

3. If there is uncertainty about the time of symptom onset, or any ongoing chest pain/discomfort or haemodynamic upset beyond 12 hours, seek advice as urgent reperfusion may still be indicated.

4. Refer to local policies for target 'call to balloon' time.

5. Thrombolytic treatment should not be regarded as the end of the emergency care of a STEMI patient. Rapid transfer to an appropriate hospital for timely therapy to prevent re-infarction, and assessment of the need for rescue PPCI, is essential.

6. Refer to reteplase or tenecteplase guidelines for the checklist to identify eligibility for prehospital thrombolysis.

Adult Bradycardia Algorithm

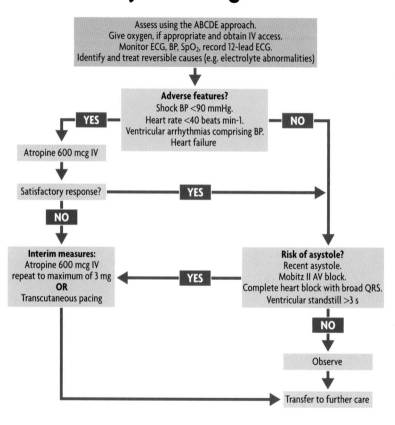

Assess using the ABCDE approach.
Give oxygen, if appropriate and obtain IV access.
Monitor ECG, BP, SpO₂, record 12-lead ECG.
Identify and treat reversible causes (e.g. electrolyte abnormalities)

Adverse features?
Shock BP <90 mmHg.
Heart rate <40 beats min-1.
Ventricular arrhythmias comprising BP.
Heart failure

YES **NO**

Atropine 600 mcg IV

Satisfactory response? **YES**

NO

Interim measures:
Atropine 600 mcg IV
repeat to maximum of 3 mg
OR
Transcutaneous pacing

YES

Risk of asystole?
Recent asystole.
Mobitz II AV block.
Complete heart block with broad QRS.
Ventricular standstill >3 s

NO

Observe

Transfer to further care

Adult Tachycardia (With Pulse)

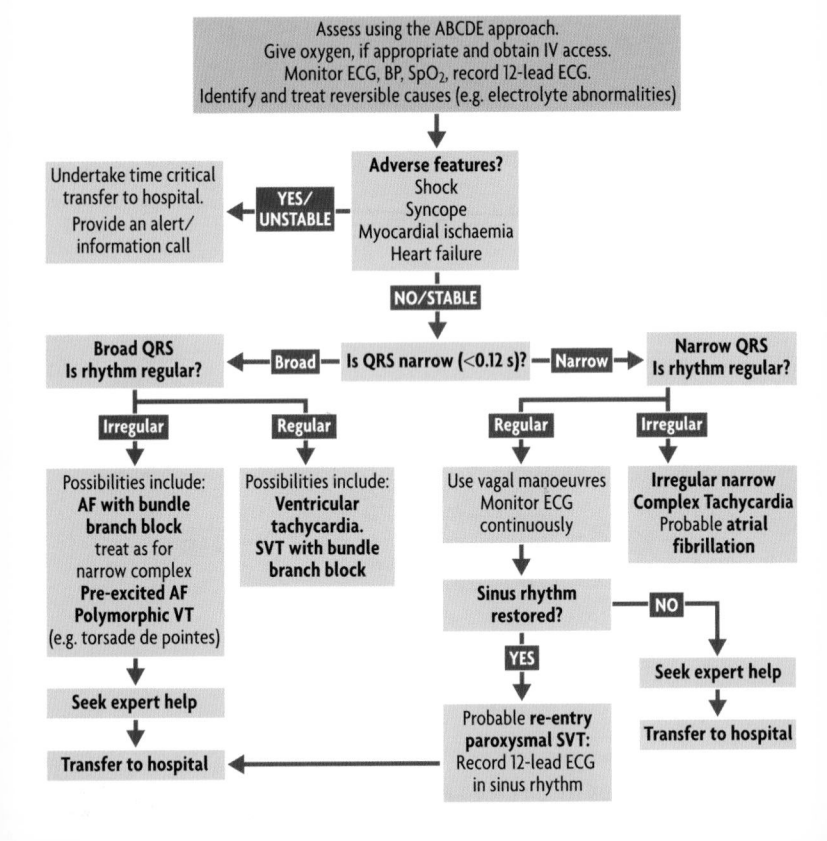

Heart Failure

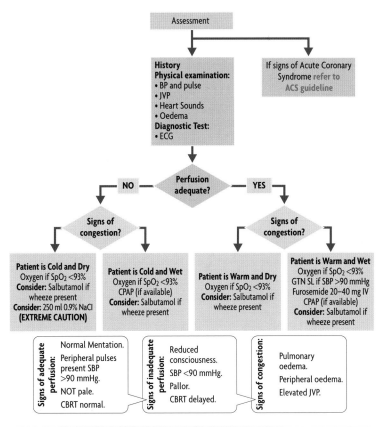

Assessment

History
Physical examination:
• BP and pulse
• JVP
• Heart Sounds
• Oedema
Diagnostic Test:
• ECG

If signs of Acute Coronary Syndrome refer to ACS guideline

Perfusion adequate?

NO — YES

Signs of congestion?

Signs of congestion?

Patient is Cold and Dry
Oxygen if SpO₂ <93%
Consider: Salbutamol if wheeze present
Consider: 250 ml 0.9% NaCl
(EXTREME CAUTION)

Patient is Cold and Wet
Oxygen if SpO₂ <93%
CPAP (if available)
Consider: Salbutamol if wheeze present

Patient is Warm and Dry
Oxygen if SpO₂ <93%
Consider: Salbutamol if wheeze present

Patient is Warm and Wet
Oxygen if SpO₂ <93%
GTN SL if SBP >90 mmHg
Furosemide 20–40 mg IV
CPAP (if available)
Consider: Salbutamol if wheeze present

Signs of adequate perfusion:
Normal Mentation.
Peripheral pulses present SBP >90 mmHg.
NOT pale.
CBRT normal.

Signs of inadequate perfusion:
Reduced consciousness.
SBP <90 mmHg.
Pallor.
CBRT delayed.

Signs of congestion:
Pulmonary oedema.
Peripheral oedema.
Elevated JVP.

Pulmonary Embolism

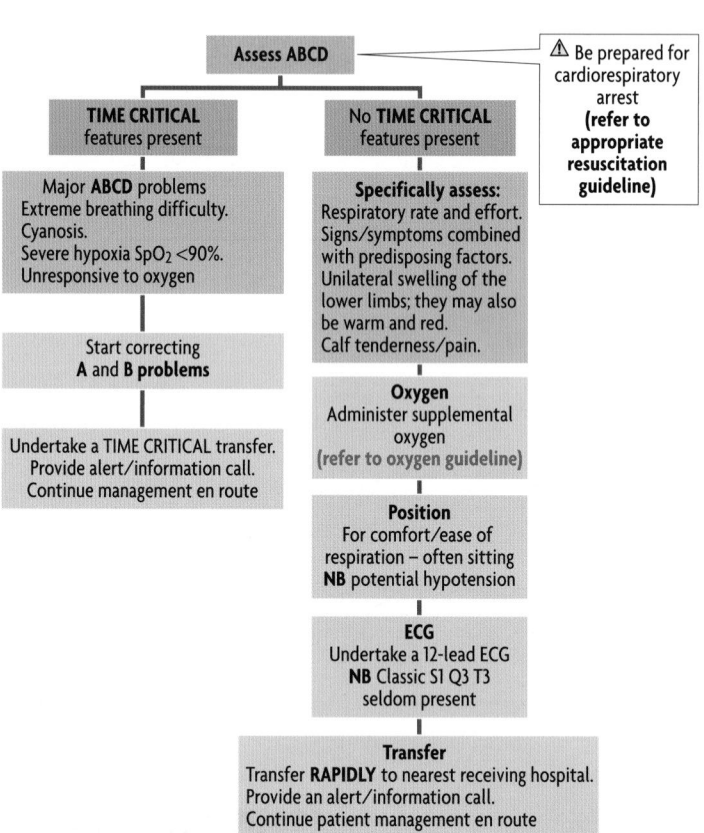

Assess ABCD

⚠ Be prepared for cardiorespiratory arrest **(refer to appropriate resuscitation guideline)**

TIME CRITICAL features present

No **TIME CRITICAL** features present

Major **ABCD** problems
Extreme breathing difficulty.
Cyanosis.
Severe hypoxia SpO$_2$ <90%.
Unresponsive to oxygen

Specifically assess:
Respiratory rate and effort.
Signs/symptoms combined with predisposing factors.
Unilateral swelling of the lower limbs; they may also be warm and red.
Calf tenderness/pain.

Start correcting **A** and **B** problems

Oxygen
Administer supplemental oxygen
(refer to oxygen guideline)

Undertake a TIME CRITICAL transfer.
Provide alert/information call.
Continue management en route

Position
For comfort/ease of respiration – often sitting
NB potential hypotension

ECG
Undertake a 12-lead ECG
NB Classic S1 Q3 T3 seldom present

Transfer
Transfer **RAPIDLY** to nearest receiving hospital.
Provide an alert/information call.
Continue patient management en route

Asthma (Adults)

MILD/ MODERATE ASTHMA	Move to a calm, quiet environment
	Encourage use of own inhaler, preferably using a spacer. Ensure correct technique is used; two puffs, followed by two puffs every 2 minutes to a maximum of ten puffs
	Administer high levels of supplementary **oxygen**
	Administer nebulised **salbutamol** using an oxygen driven nebuliser (refer to salbutamol guideline)
SEVERE ASTHMA	If no improvement, administer **ipratropium bromide** by nebuliser (refer to ipratropium bromide guideline)
	Administer steroids (refer to relevant steroids guideline)
	Continuous **salbutamol** nebulisation may be administered unless clinically significant side effects occur (refer to salbutamol guideline)
LIFE-THREATENING ASTHMA	Administer **adrenaline** (refer to adrenaline guideline)
NEAR-FATAL ASTHMA	Positive pressure nebulise using a bag-valve-mask and 'T' piece. Assess for bilateral tension pneumothorax and treat if present. Provide an alert/information call
	As you progress through the treatment algorithm consider the patient's overall response on the condition arrow and transfer as indicated

IMPROVING — CONSIDER TRANSFER

DETERIORATING — TIME CRITICAL TRANSFER

Asthma Peak Flow Charts

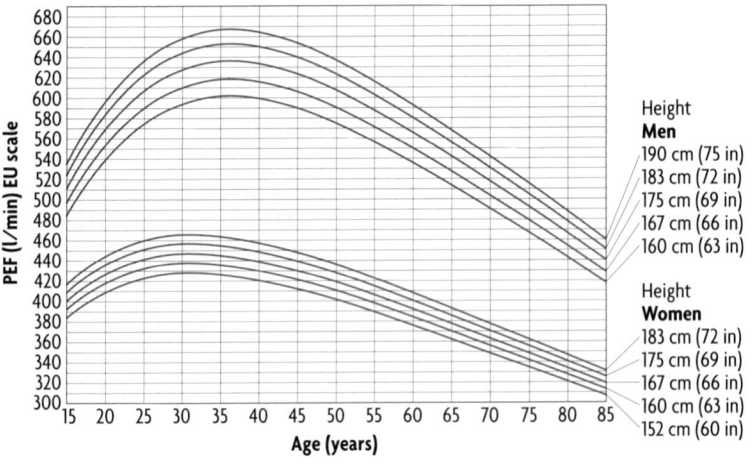

Peak flow charts – Peak expiratory flow rate – normal values. For use with EU/EN13826 scale PEF meters only.*

* Adapted by Clement Clarke for use with EN13826 / EU scale peak flow meters from Nunn AJ Gregg I, Br Med J 1989;298;1068-70.

Chronic Obstructive Pulmonary Disease

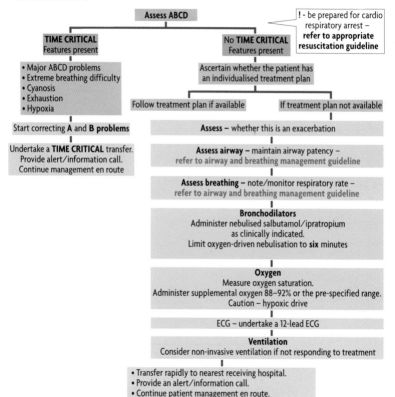

Assess ABCD

! - be prepared for cardio respiratory arrest – refer to appropriate resuscitation guideline

TIME CRITICAL Features present

No **TIME CRITICAL** Features present

- Major ABCD problems
- Extreme breathing difficulty
- Cyanosis
- Exhaustion
- Hypoxia

Ascertain whether the patient has an individualised treatment plan

Follow treatment plan if available

If treatment plan not available

Start correcting **A** and **B** problems

Undertake a **TIME CRITICAL** transfer. Provide alert/information call. Continue management en route

Assess – whether this is an exacerbation

Assess airway – maintain airway patency – refer to airway and breathing management guideline

Assess breathing – note/monitor respiratory rate – refer to airway and breathing management guideline

Bronchodilators
Administer nebulised salbutamol/ipratropium as clinically indicated.
Limit oxygen-driven nebulisation to **six** minutes

Oxygen
Measure oxygen saturation.
Administer supplemental oxygen 88–92% or the pre-specified range.
Caution – hypoxic drive

ECG – undertake a 12-lead ECG

Ventilation
Consider non-invasive ventilation if not responding to treatment

- Transfer rapidly to nearest receiving hospital.
- Provide an alert/information call.
- Continue patient management en route.
- Consider alternative care pathway where appropriate

Hyperventilation Syndrome

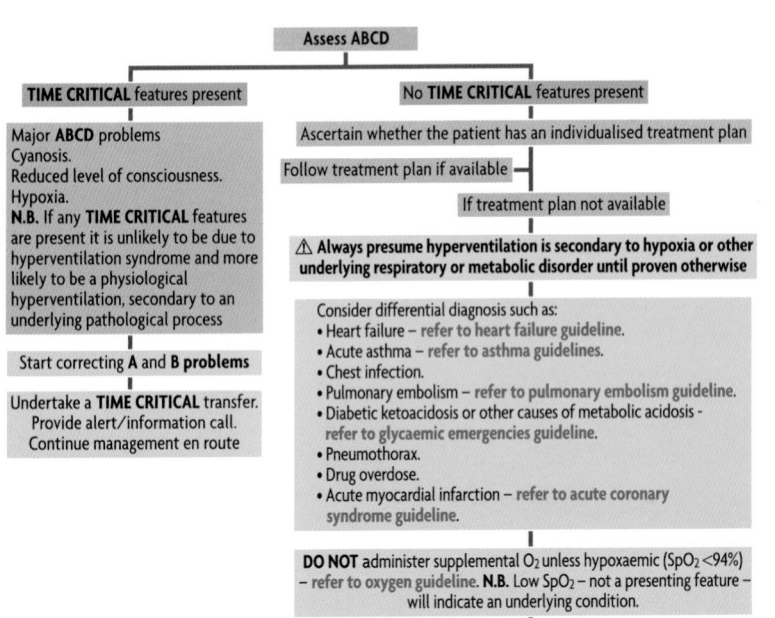

Assess ABCD

TIME CRITICAL features present

No **TIME CRITICAL** features present

Major **ABCD** problems
Cyanosis.
Reduced level of consciousness.
Hypoxia.
N.B. If any **TIME CRITICAL** features
are present it is unlikely to be due to
hyperventilation syndrome and more
likely to be a physiological
hyperventilation, secondary to an
underlying pathological process

Ascertain whether the patient has an individualised treatment plan

Follow treatment plan if available

If treatment plan not available

⚠ Always presume hyperventilation is secondary to hypoxia or other
underlying respiratory or metabolic disorder until proven otherwise

Consider differential diagnosis such as:
• Heart failure – refer to heart failure guideline.
• Acute asthma – refer to asthma guidelines.
• Chest infection.
• Pulmonary embolism – refer to pulmonary embolism guideline.
• Diabetic ketoacidosis or other causes of metabolic acidosis -
  refer to glycaemic emergencies guideline.
• Pneumothorax.
• Drug overdose.
• Acute myocardial infarction – refer to acute coronary
  syndrome guideline.

Start correcting **A** and **B** problems

Undertake a **TIME CRITICAL** transfer.
Provide alert/information call.
Continue management en route

DO NOT administer supplemental O_2 unless hypoxaemic (SpO_2 <94%)
– refer to oxygen guideline. **N.B.** Low SpO_2 – not a presenting feature –
will indicate an underlying condition.

Re-assure the patient. Coach patients regarding their respirations.
Try to remove the source of the patient's anxiety, particularly in children

Transfer to further care
Patients experiencing their first episode. Known HVS sufferers whose symptoms have not settled, or re-occur
within 10 minutes. Patients who have an individualised care plan and a responsible adult present may be
considered for non conveyance and managing at home according to local protocols.
Provide details of local care pathways if symptoms re-occur

Convulsions (Adults)

Assess ABCD

TIME CRITICAL features present

Major **ABCD** problems
Serious head injury.
Status epilepticus –
following failed treatment.
Underlying infection.
Eclampsia

Start correcting A and B problems.
Check blood glucose

Undertake a **TIME CRITICAL** transfer –
it is important to reach hospital for
definitive care as rapidly as possible –
if the patient can be transferred
despite convulsing.
Provide alert/information call.
Continue management en route

No **TIME CRITICAL features present**

Ascertain whether the patient has an individualised treatment plan

Follow treatment plan if available —— If treatment plan not available

Ascertain type of convulsion: Epileptic, Febrile, Eclamptic

Consider cause:
• **Hypoglycaemia** – check blood glucose level
  (refer to glycaemic emergencies guideline).
• **↑ Temperature** – underlying infection.
• **Head injury** – assess for signs of injury.
• **Severe hypotension** – syncope/vasovagal attack where
  patient propped up.
• **Alcohol/drug abuse.**

Monitor heart rate and rhythm

Airway
DO NOT attempt to force an oropharyngeal airway into a convulsing patient. A nasopharyngeal airway is a useful adjunct – **NB Caution in patients with suspected basal skull fracture or facial injury.**
Position patient for best airway maintenance.

Administer oxygen
Active convulsion – administer 15L per minute until a reliable SpO₂ measurement can be obtained – aim for saturation within the range of 94–98% (refer to oxygen guideline).
Post convulsion – administer supplement oxygen if hypoxaemic (SpO₂) of <94% (refer to oxygen guideline)

Medication
Establish if any treatment has been given.
Patient's own buccal midazolam for a generalised convulsion still continuing 10 minutes after the first dose of Midazolam (refer to patient's own buccal midazolam guideline).
Diazepam for fits lasting >5 minutes and **STILL FITTING**; repeated fits – not secondary to an uncorrected hypoxia or hypoglycaemic episode; status epilepticus; eclamptic fits lasting >2–3 minutes or recurrent (refer to diazepam guideline)

Transfer to further care
Patients suffering from: serial convulsions; an eclamptic convulsion ; a first convulsion; difficulties monitoring the patient's condition

Glycaemic Emergencies (Adults)

Mild	Moderate	Severe
Patient conscious, orientated and able to swallow.	Patient conscious, but confused/disorientated or aggressive and able to swallow.	Patient unconscious/convulsing or very aggressive or nil by mouth or where there is an increased risk of aspiration/choking.
Administer 15–20 grams of quick acting carbohydrate (sugary drink, chocolate bar/biscuit or glucose gel).	If capable and cooperative, administer 15–20 grams of quick acting carbohydrate (sugary drink, chocolate bar/biscuit or glucose gel). Test blood glucose level.	Assess ABCD. Measure and record blood glucose level.
Test blood glucose level if <4 mmol/L repeat up to 3 times	Continue to test after 15 minutes and repeat up to 3 times, consider intravenous glucose 10%. (Repeat up to 3 times until BGL above 4 mmol/L).	Administer IV glucose 10% by slow IV infusion (refer to glucose 10% guideline) – titrate to effect.
Consider intravenous glucose 10% or 1 mg glucagon	If NOT capable and cooperative, but able to swallow, administer 1-2 tubes of Dextrose Gel 40% or Glucagon intramuscular.	Re-assess blood glucose level after 10 minutes.
	Continue to test after 15 minutes and repeat up to 3 times, consider intravenous glucose 10%. (Repeat up to 3 times until BGL above 4 mmol/L).	If <5 mmol/L administer a further dose of IV glucose – if IV not possible administer IM glucagon (onset of action 5–10 minutes).
		Re-assess blood glucose level after a further 10 minutes.
		If no improvement transfer immediately to nearest suitable recieving hospital. Provide alert/information call.

Allergic Reactions including Anaphylaxis (Adults)

Quickly remove from trigger if possible e.g. environmental, infusion etc.
DO NOT delay definitive treatment if removing trigger not feasible

Assess ABCDE
If **TIME CRITICAL** features present – correct **A** and **B** and transfer to nearest appropriate receiving hospital. Provide an alert/information call

Consider mild/moderate allergic reaction if:
onset of illness is minutes to hours
AND
cutaneous findings e.g. urticaria
and/or angio-oedema

Consider chlorphenamine
(refer to chlorphenamine guideline)

Consider anaphylaxis if:
Sudden onset and rapid progression
Airway and/or **Breathing problems** (e.g. dyspnoea, hoarseness, stridor, wheeze, throat or chest tightness) and/or **Circulation** (e.g. hypotension, syncope, pronounced tachycardia) and/or **Skin** (e.g. erythema, urticaria, mucosal changes) problems

Administer high levels of supplementary oxygen and aim for a target saturation within the range of 94–98% (refer to oxygen guideline)

Administer adrenaline (IM only) (refer to adrenaline guideline)

If haemodynamically compromised consider fluid therapy (refer to fluid therapy guideline)

Consider chlorphenamine (refer to chlorphenamine guideline)

Consider administering hydrocortisone (refer to hydrocortisone guideline)

Consider nebulised salbutamol for bronchospasm (refer to salbutamol guideline)

Monitor and re-assess ABC.
Monitor ECG, PEFR (if possible), BP and pulse oximetry en route

Sickle Cell Crisis

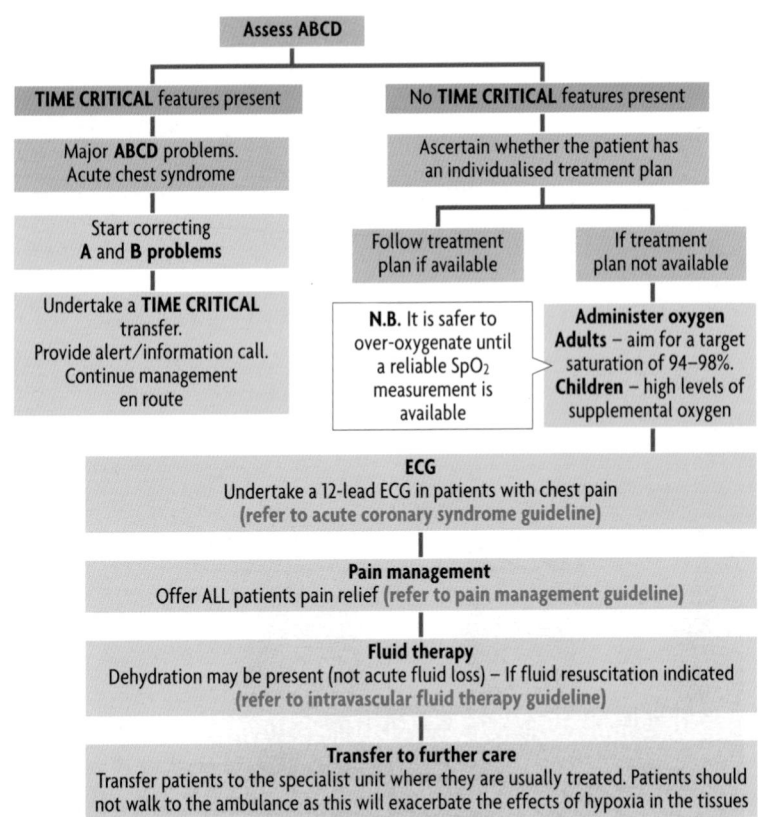

Assess ABCD

TIME CRITICAL features present

Major **ABCD** problems.
Acute chest syndrome

Start correcting
A and **B** problems

Undertake a **TIME CRITICAL**
transfer.
Provide alert/information call.
Continue management
en route

No **TIME CRITICAL** features present

Ascertain whether the patient has
an individualised treatment plan

Follow treatment
plan if available

If treatment
plan not available

N.B. It is safer to
over-oxygenate until
a reliable SpO$_2$
measurement is
available

Administer oxygen
Adults – aim for a target
saturation of 94–98%.
Children – high levels of
supplemental oxygen

ECG
Undertake a 12-lead ECG in patients with chest pain
(refer to acute coronary syndrome guideline)

Pain management
Offer ALL patients pain relief (refer to pain management guideline)

Fluid therapy
Dehydration may be present (not acute fluid loss) – If fluid resuscitation indicated
(refer to intravascular fluid therapy guideline)

Transfer to further care
Transfer patients to the specialist unit where they are usually treated. Patients should
not walk to the ambulance as this will exacerbate the effects of hypoxia in the tissues

TRAUMA

Trauma – SCENE

SCENE

S Safety

Perform a dynamic risk assessment. Are there any dangers now or will there be any that become apparent during the incident? This needs to be continually re-assessed throughout the incident. Appropriate personal protective equipment should be utilised according to local protocols.

C Cause including MOI

Establish the events leading up to the incident. Is this consistent with your findings?

E Environment

Are there any environmental factors that need to be taken into consideration? These can include problems with access or egress, weather conditions or time of day.

N Number of patients

Establish exactly how many patients there are during the initial assessment of the scene.

E Extra resources needed

Additional resources should be mobilised now. These can include additional ambulances, helicopter or senior medical support. Liaise with the major trauma advisor according to local protocols.

Trauma – ATMIST

ATMIST	
A	Age
T	Time of incident
M	Mechanism
I	Injuries
S	Signs and symptoms
T	Treatment given/immediate needs

Trauma Survey

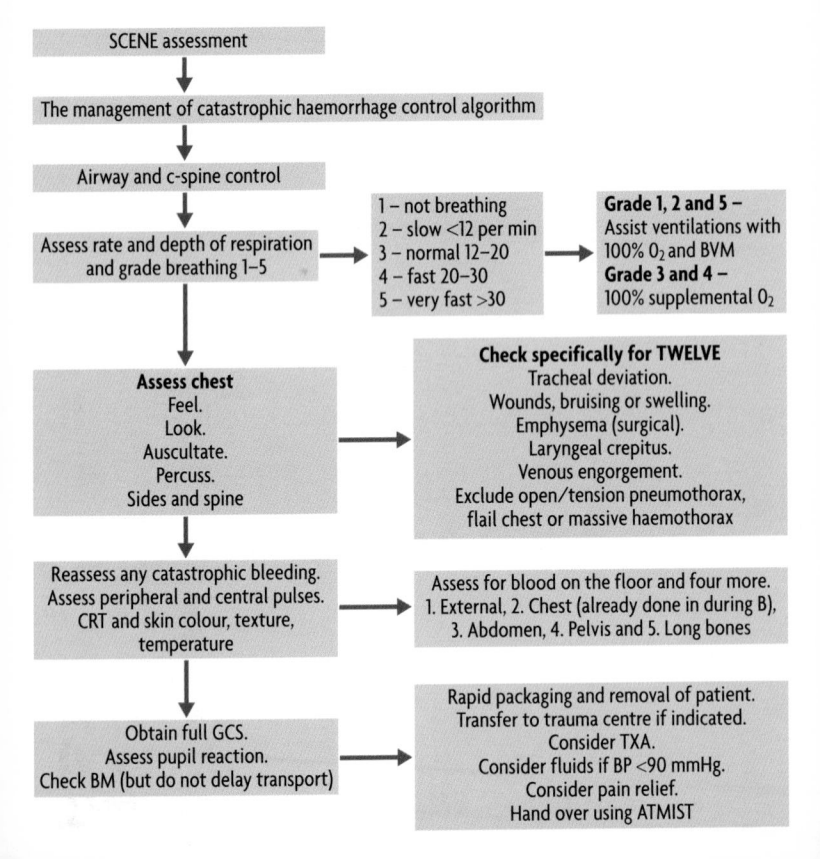

Trauma Emergencies Overview (Adults)

The management of haemorrhage algorithm.

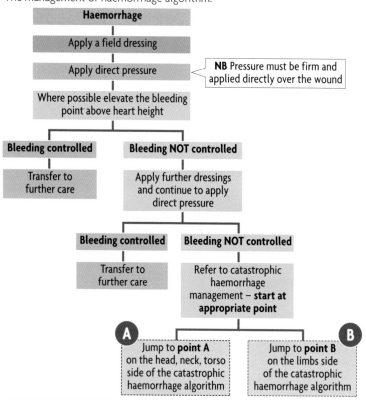

Haemorrhage

Apply a field dressing

Apply direct pressure — **NB** Pressure must be firm and applied directly over the wound

Where possible elevate the bleeding point above heart height

Bleeding controlled
Transfer to further care

Bleeding NOT controlled
Apply further dressings and continue to apply direct pressure

Bleeding controlled
Transfer to further care

Bleeding NOT controlled
Refer to catastrophic haemorrhage management – **start at appropriate point**

A Jump to **point A** on the head, neck, torso side of the catastrophic haemorrhage algorithm

B Jump to **point B** on the limbs side of the catastrophic haemorrhage algorithm

Trauma Emergencies Overview (Adults)

The management of catastrophic haemorrhage algorithm.

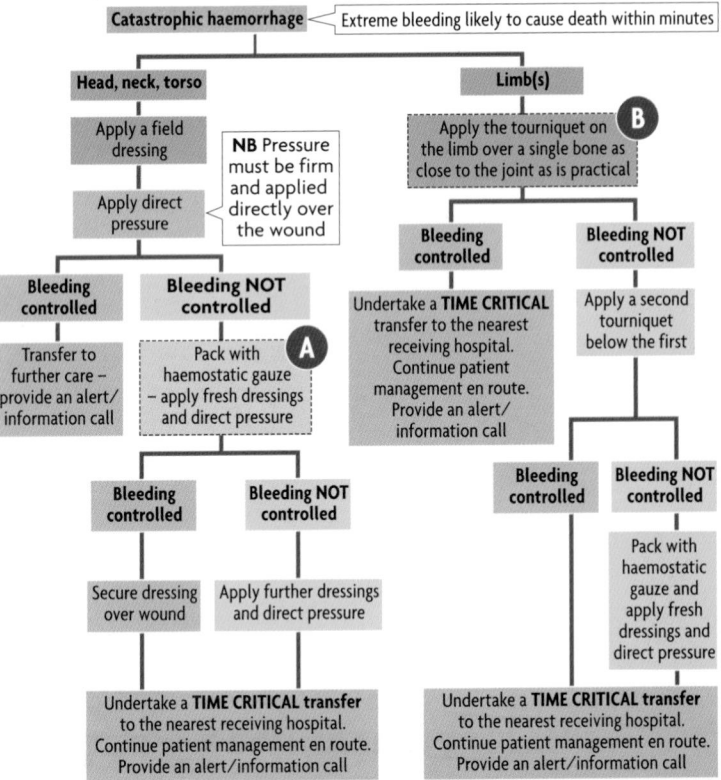

Neck and Back Trauma

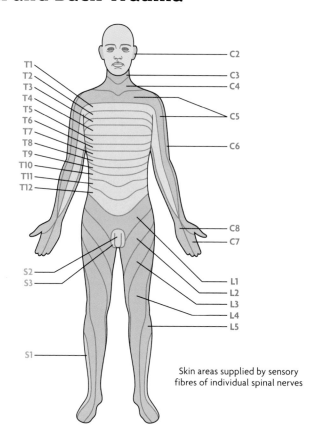

Skin areas supplied by sensory fibres of individual spinal nerves

Neck and Back Trauma

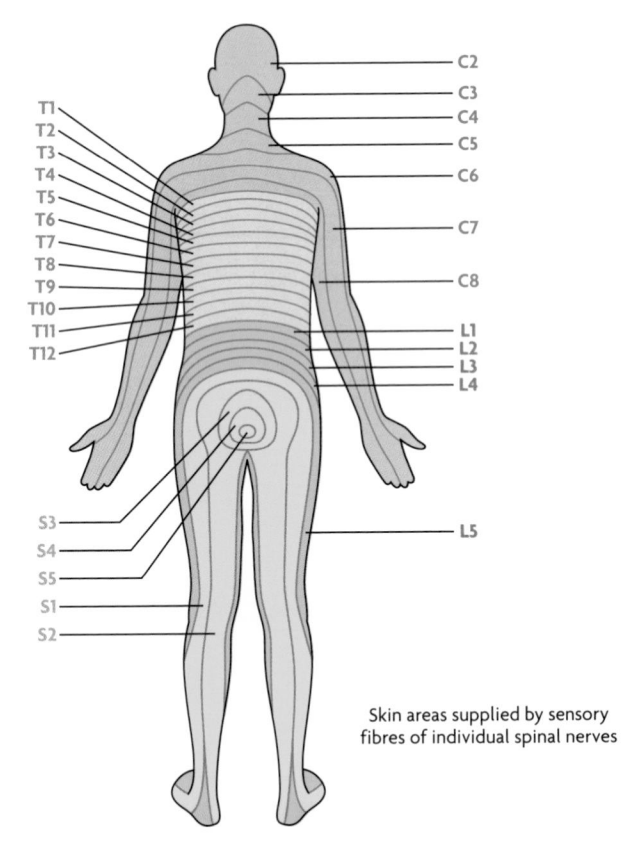

Skin areas supplied by sensory fibres of individual spinal nerves

Neck and Back Trauma

Immobilisation algorithm.

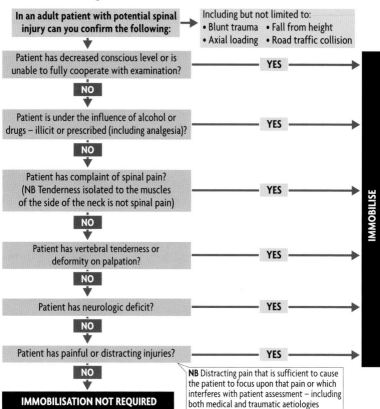

In an adult patient with potential spinal injury can you confirm the following:

Including but not limited to:
- Blunt trauma
- Axial loading
- Fall from height
- Road traffic collision

Patient has decreased conscious level or is unable to fully cooperate with examination? **YES** → IMMOBILISE

NO

Patient is under the influence of alcohol or drugs – illicit or prescribed (including analgesia)? **YES** → IMMOBILISE

NO

Patient has complaint of spinal pain? (NB Tenderness isolated to the muscles of the side of the neck is not spinal pain) **YES** → IMMOBILISE

NO

Patient has vertebral tenderness or deformity on palpation? **YES** → IMMOBILISE

NO

Patient has neurologic deficit? **YES** → IMMOBILISE

NO

Patient has painful or distracting injuries? **YES** → IMMOBILISE

NO

IMMOBILISATION NOT REQUIRED

NB Distracting pain that is sufficient to cause the patient to focus upon that pain or which interferes with patient assessment – including both medical and traumatic aetiologies

Intravascular Fluid Therapy (Adults)

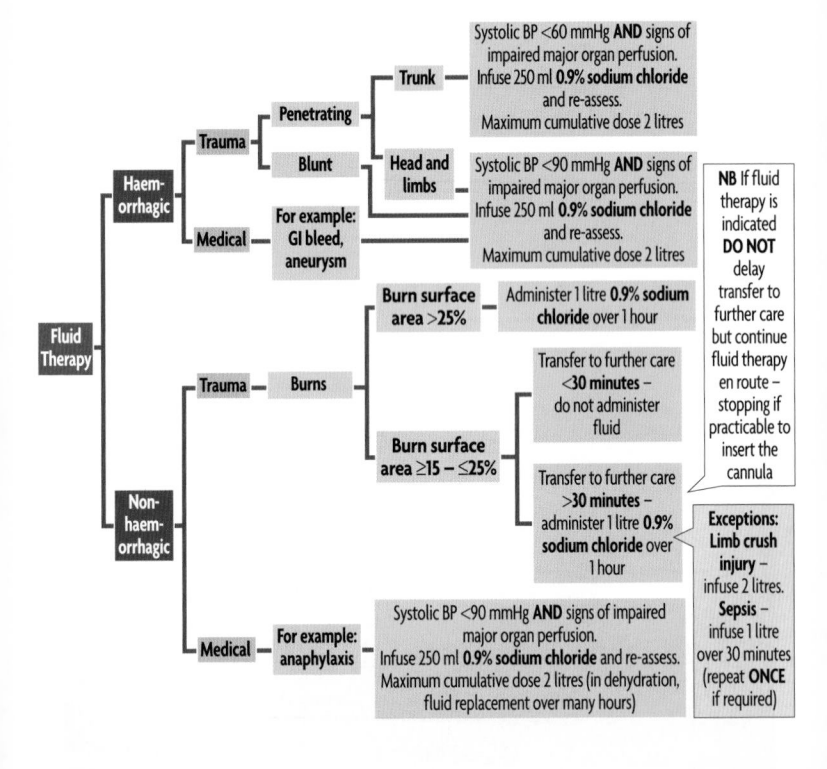

Fluid Therapy

Haemorrhagic

Trauma

Penetrating — **Trunk**
Systolic BP <60 mmHg **AND** signs of impaired major organ perfusion. Infuse 250 ml **0.9% sodium chloride** and re-assess. Maximum cumulative dose 2 litres

Blunt — **Head and limbs**
Systolic BP <90 mmHg **AND** signs of impaired major organ perfusion. Infuse 250 ml **0.9% sodium chloride** and re-assess. Maximum cumulative dose 2 litres

Medical — For example: GI bleed, aneurysm

NB If fluid therapy is indicated **DO NOT** delay transfer to further care but continue fluid therapy en route – stopping if practicable to insert the cannula

Non-haemorrhagic

Trauma — **Burns**

Burn surface area >25%
Administer 1 litre **0.9% sodium chloride** over 1 hour

Burn surface area ≥15 – ≤25%
Transfer to further care <30 minutes – do not administer fluid

Transfer to further care >30 minutes – administer 1 litre **0.9% sodium chloride** over 1 hour

Exceptions: Limb crush injury – infuse 2 litres. **Sepsis** – infuse 1 litre over 30 minutes (repeat **ONCE** if required)

Medical — For example: anaphylaxis
Systolic BP <90 mmHg **AND** signs of impaired major organ perfusion. Infuse 250 ml **0.9% sodium chloride** and re-assess. Maximum cumulative dose 2 litres (in dehydration, fluid replacement over many hours)

SPECIAL
SITUATIONS

METHANE Report Format

METHANE Report Format	
M	Major incident standby or declared
E	Exact location of incident
T	Type of incident
H	Hazards (present and potential)
A	Access and egress routes
N	Number, severity and type of casualties
E	Emergency services present on scene and further resources required

Triage Model

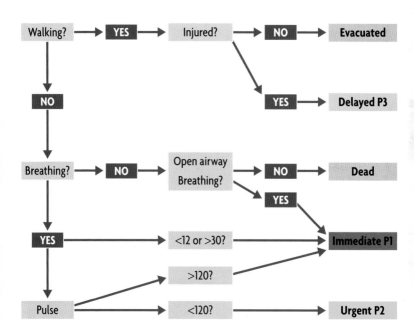

Chemical, Biological, Radiological, Nuclear and Explosive Incidents

General management for an unspecified CBRNE incident.

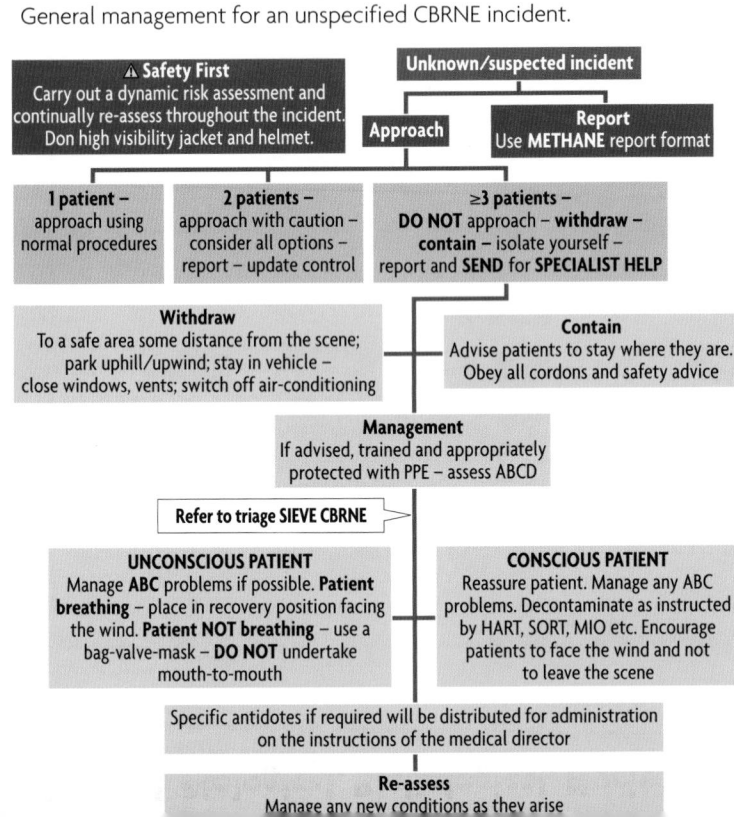

Chemical, Biological, Radiological, Nuclear and Explosive Incidents — continued from page 44

CBRNE (SPECIAL AGENT) TRIAGE SIEVE: For use before and during decontamination.

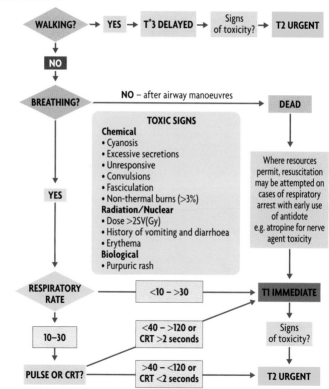

* In this guideline the letter 'T' stands for triage, but in some documents 'P' may be used, which stands for priority; these terms are interchangeable.

WALKING? → YES → T*3 DELAYED → Signs of toxicity? → T2 URGENT

NO

BREATHING? → NO – after airway manoeuvres → DEAD

Where resources permit, resuscitation may be attempted on cases of respiratory arrest with early use of antidote e.g. atropine for nerve agent toxicity

YES

TOXIC SIGNS
Chemical
• Cyanosis
• Excessive secretions
• Unresponsive
• Convulsions
• Fasciculation
• Non-thermal burns (>3%)
Radiation/Nuclear
• Dose >2SV(Gy)
• History of vomiting and diarrhoea
• Erythema
Biological
• Purpuric rash

RESPIRATORY RATE → <10 - >30 → T1 IMMEDIATE

10–30

PULSE OR CRT? → <40 - >120 or CRT >2 seconds → T1 IMMEDIATE → Signs of toxicity? → T2 URGENT

>40 - <120 or CRT <2 seconds → T2 URGENT

PAEDIATRICS

Basic Life Support (Child)

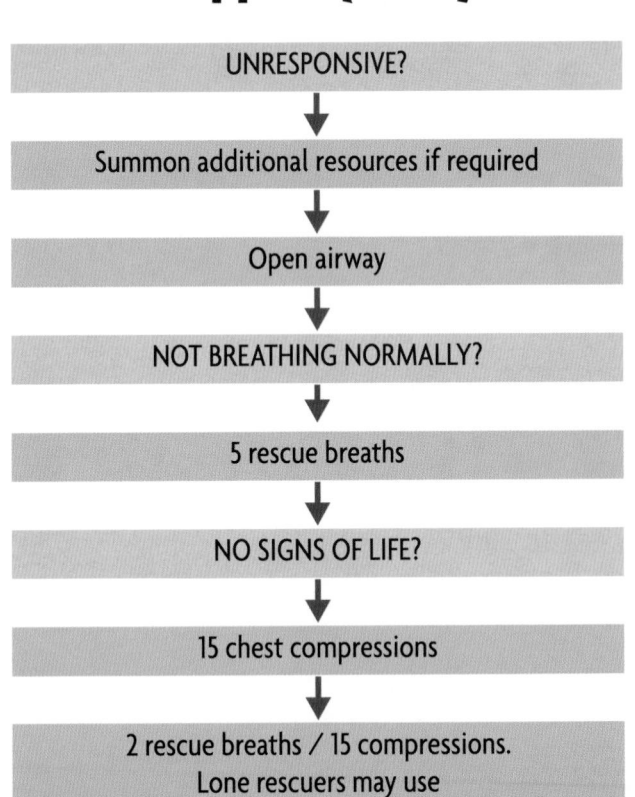

UNRESPONSIVE?

↓

Summon additional resources if required

↓

Open airway

↓

NOT BREATHING NORMALLY?

↓

5 rescue breaths

↓

NO SIGNS OF LIFE?

↓

15 chest compressions

↓

2 rescue breaths / 15 compressions.
Lone rescuers may use
2 rescue breaths / 30 compressions

Advanced Life Support (Child)

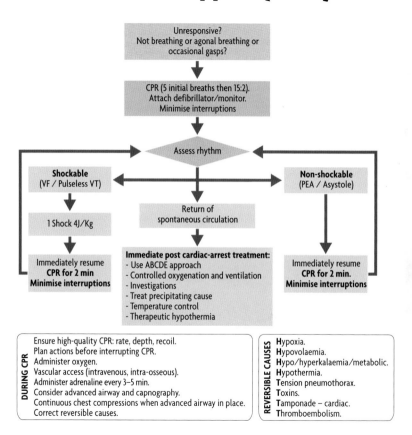

Unresponsive?
Not breathing or agonal breathing or
occasional gasps?

↓

CPR (5 initial breaths then 15:2).
Attach defibrillator/monitor.
Minimise interruptions

↓

Assess rhythm

Shockable
(VF / Pulseless VT)

↓

1 Shock 4J/Kg

↓

Immediately resume
**CPR for 2 min
Minimise interruptions**

Return of
spontaneous circulation

↓

Immediate post cardiac-arrest treatment:
- Use ABCDE approach
- Controlled oxygenation and ventilation
- Investigations
- Treat precipitating cause
- Temperature control
- Therapeutic hypothermia

Non-shockable
(PEA / Asystole)

↓

Immediately resume
**CPR for 2 min.
Minimise interruptions**

DURING CPR
Ensure high-quality CPR: rate, depth, recoil.
Plan actions before interrupting CPR.
Administer oxygen.
Vascular access (intravenous, intra-osseous).
Administer adrenaline every 3–5 min.
Consider advanced airway and capnography.
Continuous chest compressions when advanced airway in place.
Correct reversible causes.

REVERSIBLE CAUSES
Hypoxia.
Hypovolaemia.
Hypo/hyperkalaemia/metabolic.
Hypothermia.
Tension pneumothorax.
Toxins.
Tamponade – cardiac.
Thromboembolism.

Newborn Life Support

Dry the baby
Remove any wet towels and cover.
Start the clock or note the time

Birth

↓

Assess (tone)
Breathing and heart rate

30 sec

60 sec

↓

If gasping or not breathing
Open the airway. Give 5 inflation breaths. Consider SpO2

↓

Re-assess
If no increase in heart rate look for chest movement

↓

If chest not moving:
Recheck head position.
Consider 2-person airway control and other airway manoeuvres.
Repeat inflation breaths.
Consider SpO2. Look for a response

↓

If no increase in heart rate look for chest movement

↓

When the chest is moving:
If heart rate is not detectable or slow (<60)
Start chest compressions – 3 compressions to each breath

↓

Re-assess heart rate every 30 seconds.
Undertake a **TIME CRITICAL** transfer immediately.
Provide an alert/information call

AT ALL STAGES ASK: DO I NEED HELP?

Acceptable SpO2

2 min	60%
3 min	70%
4 min	80%
5 min	85%
10 min	90%

Foreign Body Airway Obstruction

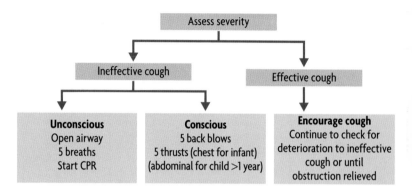

Assess severity

Ineffective cough

Unconscious
Open airway
5 breaths
Start CPR

Conscious
5 back blows
5 thrusts (chest for infant)
(abdominal for child >1 year)

Effective cough

Encourage cough
Continue to check for
deterioration to ineffective
cough or until
obstruction relieved

Death of a Child, including Sudden Unexpected Death in Infancy, Children and Adolescents (SUDICA)

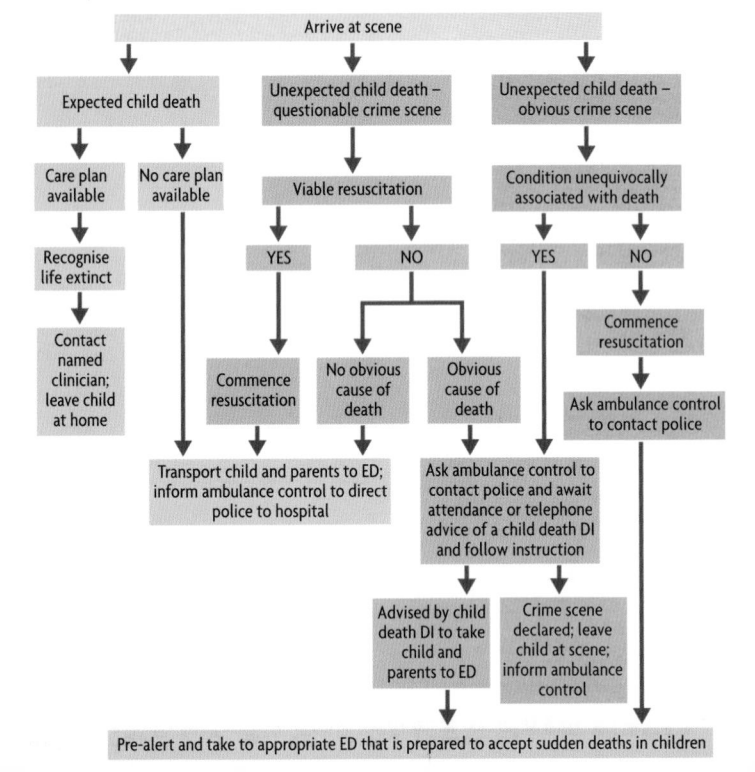

The Wong-Baker FACES Pain Rating Scale

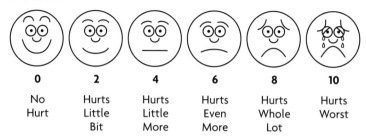

0	2	4	6	8	10
No Hurt	Hurts Little Bit	Hurts Little More	Hurts Even More	Hurts Whole Lot	Hurts Worst

This rating scale is recommended for persons aged 3 years and older.

Instructions: Point to each face using the words to describe the pain intensity. Ask the child to choose face that best describes own pain and record the appropriate number.

Explain to the person that each face is for a person who feels happy because he has no pain (hurt) or sad because he has some or a lot of pain.

Face 0 is very happy because he doesn't hurt at all.
Face 2 hurts just a little bit.
Face 4 hurts a little more.
Face 6 hurts even more.
Face 8 hurts a whole lot.
Face 10 hurts as much as you can imagine, although you don't have to be crying to feel this bad.

Ask the person to choose the face that best describes how they are feeling.

From Hockenberry MJ, Wilson D, Winkelstein ML: Wong's Essentials of Pediatric Nursing, ed. 7, St. Louis, 2005, p. 1259. Used with permission. Copyright, Mosby.

The FLACC Scale

The **Face, Legs, Activity, Cry, Consolability scale** or **FLACC scale** is a measurement used to assess pain for children up to the age of 7 years or individuals who are unable to communicate their pain. The scale is scored on a range of 0–10 with 0 representing no pain. The scale has five criteria which are each assigned a score of 0, 1 or 2.

Criteria	Score - 0	Score - 1	Score - 2
Face	No particular expression or smile	Occasional grimace or frown, withdrawn, uninterested	Frequent to constant quivering chin, clenched jaw
Legs	Normal position or relaxed	Uneasy, restless, tense	Kicking, or legs drawn up
Activity	Lying quietly, normal position, moves easily	Squirming, shifting back and forth, tense	Arched, rigid or jerking
Cry	No cry (awake or asleep)	Moans or whimpers, occasional complaint	Crying steadily, screams or sobs, frequent complaints
Consolability	Content, relaxed	Reassured by occasional touching, hugging or being talked to, distractible	Difficult to console or comfort

GREEN: NICE 'Traffic Lights' Clinical Assessment Tool for Febrile Illness in Children

Colour	Normal colour of skin, lips and tongue
Activity	Responds normally to social cues Content/smiles Stays awake or awakens quickly Strong/normal cry/not crying
Hydration	Normal skin and eyes Moist mucous membranes
Other	No amber or red symptoms or signs

AMBER: NICE 'Traffic Lights' Clinical Assessment Tool for Febrile Illness in Children

Colour	Pallor reported by parent/carer
Activity	Not responding normally to social cues Wakes only with prolonged stimulation Decreased activity No smile

Respiratory	Nasal flaring
	Tachypnoea:
	  ● RR >50/min age 6–12 months
	  ● RR >40/min age >12 months
	O_2 sats ≤ 95% in air
	Crackles

Hydration	Dry mucous membranes Poor feeding in infants Capillary Refill Time (CRT) ≥3 seconds ↓Urinary output
Other	Fever for ≥5 days Swelling of a limb or joint Non-weight bearing/not using an extremity A new lump >2 cm

RED: NICE 'Traffic Lights' Clinical Assessment Tool for Febrile Illness in Children

Colour	Pale/mottled/ashen/blue
Activity	No response to social cues Appears ill to a healthcare professional Unable to rouse, or if roused, does not stay awake Weak/high pitched/continuous cry
Respiratory	Grunting Tachypnoea: RR >60/min Moderate or severe chest indrawing
Hydration	Reduced skin turgor
Other	0-3 months, temp ≥38°C 3–6 months, temp ≥39°C Non-blanching rash Bulging fontanelle Neck stiffness Status epilepticus Focal seizures Focal neurological signs Bile-stained vomiting

Modified Taussig Croup Score

		Score*
Stridor	None	0
	Only on crying, exertion	1
	At rest	2
	Severe (biphasic)	3
Recession	None	0
	Only on crying, exertion	1
	At rest	2
	Severe (biphasic)	3

* Mild: 1–2; Moderate: 3–4; Severe: 5–6

Meningococcal Meningitis and Septicaemia

Management algorithm for patients with suspected meningococcal disease.

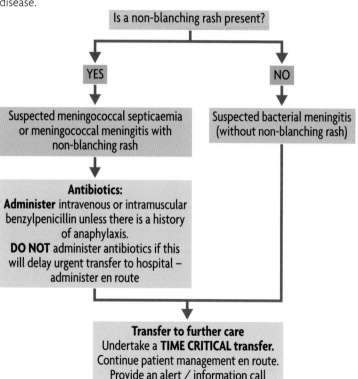

Is a non-blanching rash present?

YES

NO

Suspected meningococcal septicaemia or meningococcal meningitis with non-blanching rash

Suspected bacterial meningitis (without non-blanching rash)

Antibiotics:
Administer intravenous or intramuscular benzylpenicillin unless there is a history of anaphylaxis.
DO NOT administer antibiotics if this will delay urgent transfer to hospital – administer en route

Transfer to further care
Undertake a **TIME CRITICAL** transfer.
Continue patient management en route.
Provide an alert / information call

Allergic Reactions including Anaphylaxis (Children)

Quickly remove from trigger if possible e.g. environmental, infusion etc.
DO NOT delay definitive treatment if removing trigger not feasible

Assess ABCDE
If TIME CRITICAL features present – correct A and B and transfer to nearest suitable receiving hospital. Provide an alert/information call

Consider mild/moderate allergic reaction if:
Onset of illness is minutes to hours
AND
Cutaneous findings e.g. urticaria and/or angio-oedema

Consider chlorphenamine
(refer to chlorphenamine guideline)

Consider anaphylaxis if:
Sudden onset and rapid progression
Airway and/or **Breathing** problems (e.g. dyspnoea, hoarseness, stridor, wheeze, throat or chest tightness) and/or **Circulation** (e.g. hypotension, syncope, pronounced tachycardia) and/or **Skin** (e.g. erythema, urticaria, mucosal changes) problems

Administer high levels of supplementary oxygen
(refer to oxygen guideline)

Administer adrenaline 1 in 1000 IM only
(refer to adrenaline guideline)

If haemodynamically compromised
(refer to intravenous fluid therapy guideline)

Consider chlorphenamine
(refer to chlorphenamine guideline)

Consider administering hydrocortisone
(refer to hydrocortisone guideline)

Consider nebulised salbutamol for bronchospasm
(refer to salbutamol guideline)

Monitor and re-assess ABC
Monitor ECG, PEFR (If possible), BP and pulse oximetry en route

Asthma (Children)

Asthma assessment and management algorithm.

MILD/ MODERATE ASTHMA

Move to a calm, quiet environment

Encourage use of own inhaler, preferably using a spacer. Ensure correct technique is used; two puffs, followed by two puffs every 2 minutes to a maximum of ten puffs

Administer high levels of supplementary **oxygen**

Administer nebulised **salbutamol** using an oxygen driven nebuliser (refer to salbutamol guideline)

SEVERE ASTHMA

If no improvement, administer **ipratropium bromide** by nebuliser (refer to ipratropium bromide guideline)

Administer steroids (refer to relevant steroids guideline)

Continuous **salbutamol** nebulisation may be administered unless clinically significant side effects occur (refer to salbutamol guideline)

LIFE-THREATENING ASTHMA

Administer **adrenaline** (refer to adrenaline guideline) NB Check child is still receiving high levels of oxygen before administering

NEAR-FATAL ASTHMA

Positive pressure nebulise using a bag-valve-mask and 'T' piece. Provide an alert/information call

As you progress through the treatment algorithm consider the patient's overall response on the condition arrow and transfer as indicated

IMPROVING | CONSIDER TRANSFER

DETERIORATING | TIME CRITICAL TRANSFER

Peak Expiratory Flow Chart

Height (m)	Height (ft)	Predicted EU PEFR (L/min)
0.85	2'9"	87
0.90	2'11"	95
0.95	3'1"	104
1.00	3'3"	115
1.05	3'5"	127
1.10	3'7"	141
1.15	3'9"	157
1.20	3'11"	174
1.25	4'1"	192
1.30	4'3"	212
1.35	4'5"	233
1.40	4'7"	254
1.45	4'9"	276
1.50	4'11"	299
1.55	5'1"	323
1.60	5'3"	346
1.65	5'5"	370
1.70	5'7"	393

Convulsions (Children)

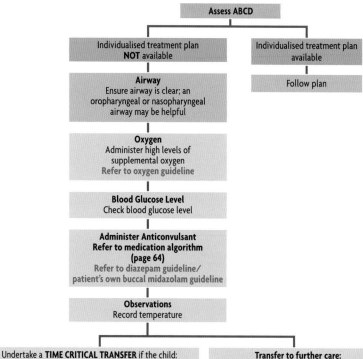

Assess ABCD

Individualised treatment plan NOT available

Airway
Ensure airway is clear; an oropharyngeal or nasopharyngeal airway may be helpful

Oxygen
Administer high levels of supplemental oxygen
Refer to oxygen guideline

Blood Glucose Level
Check blood glucose level

Administer Anticonvulsant
Refer to medication algorithm (page 64)
Refer to diazepam guideline/ patient's own buccal midazolam guideline

Observations
Record temperature

Individualised treatment plan available

Follow plan

Undertake a **TIME CRITICAL TRANSFER** if the child:
• is still convulsing
• is in status epilepticus
• has suspected meningococcal septicaemia or meningitis.
Provide an **alert/information call**

Transfer to further care:
• Children <2 year old.
• Children with a febrile convulsion.
• Children receiving >1 dose of anticonvulsant.
• Children who have not yet fully recovered

Convulsions (Children)

Medication algorithm for convulsions in children.

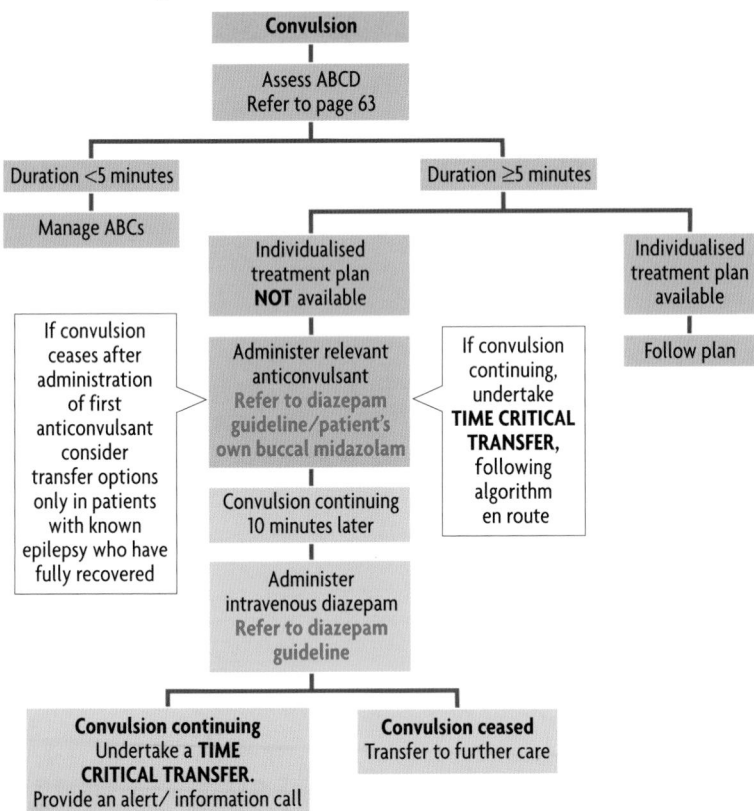

Trauma Emergencies Overview (Children)

The management of haemorrhage algorithm.

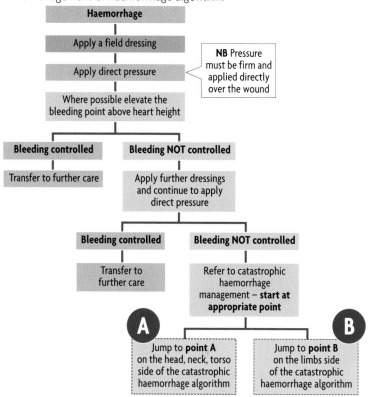

Haemorrhage

Apply a field dressing

Apply direct pressure

NB Pressure must be firm and applied directly over the wound

Where possible elevate the bleeding point above heart height

Bleeding controlled

Transfer to further care

Bleeding NOT controlled

Apply further dressings and continue to apply direct pressure

Bleeding controlled

Transfer to further care

Bleeding NOT controlled

Refer to catastrophic haemorrhage management – **start at appropriate point**

A

Jump to **point A** on the head, neck, torso side of the catastrophic haemorrhage algorithm

B

Jump to **point B** on the limbs side of the catastrophic haemorrhage algorithm

Trauma Emergencies Overview (Children)

The management of catastrophic haemorrhage algorithm.

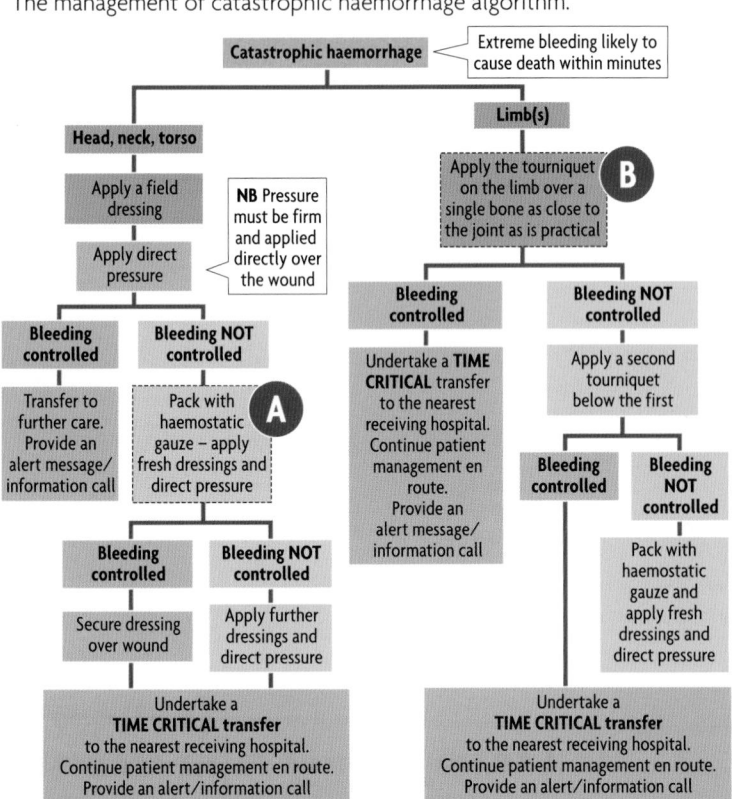

Intravascular Fluid Therapy (Children)

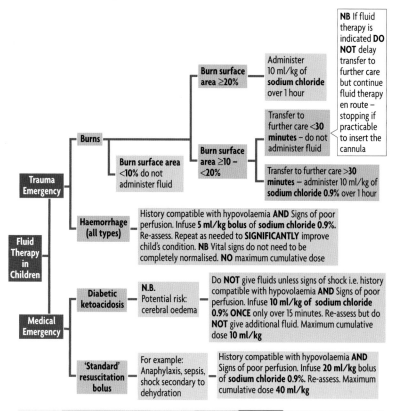

NB If fluid therapy is indicated **DO NOT** delay transfer to further care but continue fluid therapy en route – stopping if practicable to insert the cannula

Fluid Therapy in Children

Trauma Emergency

Burns

Burn surface area ≥20%
Administer 10 ml/kg of **sodium chloride** over 1 hour

Burn surface area <10% do not administer fluid

Burn surface area ≥10 – <20%
Transfer to further care **<30 minutes** – do not administer fluid

Transfer to further care **>30 minutes** – administer 10 ml/kg of **sodium chloride 0.9%** over 1 hour

Haemorrhage (all types)
History compatible with hypovolaemia **AND** Signs of poor perfusion. Infuse **5 ml/kg bolus** of **sodium chloride 0.9%**. Re-assess. Repeat as needed to **SIGNIFICANTLY** improve child's condition. **NB** Vital signs do not need to be completely normalised. **NO** maximum cumulative dose

Medical Emergency

Diabetic ketoacidosis
N.B. Potential risk: cerebral oedema

Do **NOT** give fluids unless signs of shock i.e. history compatible with hypovolaemia **AND** Signs of poor perfusion. Infuse **10 ml/kg of sodium chloride 0.9% ONCE** only over 15 minutes. Re-assess but do **NOT** give additional fluid. Maximum cumulative dose **10 ml/kg**

'Standard' resuscitation bolus
For example: Anaphylaxis, sepsis, shock secondary to dehydration

History compatible with hypovolaemia **AND** Signs of poor perfusion. Infuse **20 ml/kg bolus** of **sodium chloride 0.9%**. Re-assess. Maximum cumulative dose **40 ml/kg**

DRUGS

Adrenaline

Presentation

Pre-filled syringe or ampoule containing 1 milligram of adrenaline (epinephrine) in 1 ml (1:1,000) ADM.

Pre-filled syringe containing 1 milligram of adrenaline (epinephrine) in 10 ml (1:10,000) ADX.

Indications

Cardiac arrest.

Anaphylaxis.

Life-threatening asthma with failing ventilation and continued deterioration despite nebuliser therapy.

Actions

Adrenaline is a sympathomimetic that stimulates both alpha- and beta-adrenergic receptors. As a result myocardial and cerebral blood flow is enhanced during CPR and CPR becomes more effective due to increased peripheral resistance which improves perfusion pressures.

Reverses allergic manifestations of acute anaphylaxis.

Relieves bronchospasm in acute severe asthma.

Contra-indications

Do not give repeated doses of adrenaline in hypothermic patients.

Adrenaline

Cautions

Severe hypertension may occur in patients on beta-blockers and half doses should be administered unless there is profound hypotension.

Dosage and Administration

1. **Cardiac arrest:**

● **Shockable rhythms:** administer adrenaline after the 3rd shock and then after alternate shocks i.e. 5th, 7th etc.

● **Non-shockable rhythms:** administer adrenaline immediately IV access is achieved then alternate loops.

Route: Intravenous/intra-osseous – **administer as a rapid bolus**.

AGE	INITIAL DOSE	REPEAT DOSE	DOSE INTERVAL	VOLUME	MAXIMUM DOSE
Adult 1 milligram in 10 ml (1:10,000)	1 milligram	1 milligram	3–5 mins	10 ml	No limit

Adrenaline

2. **Anaphylaxis** and **life-threatening asthma.**

Route: Intramuscular – antero-lateral aspect of thigh or upper arm.

AGE	INITIAL DOSE	REPEAT DOSE	DOSE INTERVAL	VOLUME	MAXIMUM DOSE
Adult 1 milligram in 1 ml (1:1,000)	500 micrograms	500 micrograms	5 mins	0.5 ml	No limit

Amiodarone

AMO

Presentation

Pre-filled syringe containing 300 milligrams amiodarone in 10 ml.

Indications

Cardiac arrest

● **Shockable rhythms:** if unresponsive to defibrillation administer
amiodarone after the 3rd shock and an additional bolus depending
on age to unresponsive VF or pulseless VT following the 5th shock.

Actions

Antiarrhythmic; lengthens cardiac action potential and therefore
effective refractory period. Prolongs QT interval on ECG.

Blocks sodium and potassium channels in cardiac muscle.

Acts to stabilise and reduce electrical irritability of cardiac muscle.

Contra-indications

**No contra-indications in the context of the treatment of cardiac
arrest.**

Side Effects

Bradycardia.

Vasodilatation causing hypotension, flushing.

Bronchospasm.

Arrhythmias – Torsades de pointes.

Amiodarone

AMO

Dosage and Administration

- Administer into large vein as extravasation can cause burns.
- Follow administration with a 0.9% sodium chloride flush – **refer to sodium chloride guideline**.
- Cardiac arrest – Shockable rhythms: if unresponsive to defibrillation administer amiodarone after the 3rd and 5th shock.

Route: intravenous/intra-osseous – administer as a rapid bolus.

AGE	INITIAL DOSE	REPEAT DOSE	DOSE INTERVAL	VOLUME	MAXIMUM DOSE
Adult 300 milligrams in 10 ml	300 milligrams	150 milligrams	After 5th shock	10 ml	450 milligrams

Aspirin

Presentation

300 milligram aspirin (acetylsalicylic acid) in tablet form (dispersible).

Indications

Adults with:

● Clinical or ECG evidence suggestive of myocardial infarction or ischaemia.

Actions

Has an anti-platelet action which reduces clot formation.

Analgesic, anti-pyretic and anti-inflammatory.

Contra-indications

● Known aspirin allergy or sensitivity.

● Children under 16 years (see additional information).

● Active gastrointestinal bleeding.

● Haemophilia or other known clotting disorders.

● Severe hepatic disease.

Cautions

As the likely benefits of a single 300 milligram aspirin outweigh the potential risks, aspirin may be given to patients with:

● Asthma.

● Pregnancy.

● Kidney or liver failure.

Aspirin

ASP

- Gastric or duodenal ulcer.
- Current treatment with anticoagulants.

Side Effects

- Gastric bleeding.
- Wheezing in some asthmatics.

Additional Information

In suspected myocardial infarction a 300 milligram aspirin tablet should be given regardless of any previous aspirin taken that day.

Clopidogrel may be indicated in acute ST segment elevation myocardial infarction – **refer to clopidogrel guideline**.

Aspirin is contra-indicated in children under the age of 16 years as it may precipitate Reye's Syndrome. This syndrome is very rare and occurs in young children, damaging the liver and brain. It has a mortality rate of 50%.

Dosage and Administration

Route: Oral – chewed or dissolved in water.

AGE	INITIAL DOSE	REPEAT DOSE	DOSE INTERVAL	VOLUME	MAXIMUM DOSE
Adult 300 milligrams	300 milligrams	NONE	N/A	1 tablet	300 milligrams

Atropine

Presentation

Pre-filled syringe containing 1 milligram atropine in 10 ml.

Pre-filled syringe containing 1 milligram atropine in 5 ml.

Pre-filled syringe containing 3 milligrams atropine in 10 ml.

An ampoule containing 600 micrograms in 1 ml.

Indications

Symptomatic bradycardia in the presence of **ANY** of these adverse signs:
- Absolute bradycardia (pulse <40 beats per minute).
- Systolic blood pressure below expected for age (**refer to page for age guideline** for age related blood pressure readings in children).
- Paroxysmal ventricular arrhythmias requiring suppression.
- Inadequate perfusion causing confusion etc.

NB Hypoxia is the most common cause of bradycardia in children, therefore interventions to support ABC and oxygen therapy should be the first-line therapy.

Contra-indications

Should **NOT** be given to treat bradycardia in suspected hypothermia.

Actions

May reverse effects of vagal overdrive.

May increase heart rate by blocking vagal activity in sinus bradycardia, second or third degree heart block.

Enhances A-V conduction.

Atropine

ATR

Side Effects

Dry mouth, visual blurring and pupil dilation.

Confusion and occasional hallucinations.

Tachycardia.

In the elderly retention of urine may occur.

Do not use small (<100 micrograms) doses as they may cause paradoxical bradycardia.

Additional Information

May induce tachycardia when used after myocardial infarction, which will increase myocardial oxygen demand and worsen ischaemia. Hence, bradycardia in a patient with an MI should **ONLY** be treated if the low heart rate is causing problems with perfusion, such as hypotension.

Dosage and Administration

SYMPTOMATIC BRADYCARDIA

NB BRADYCARDIA in children is most commonly caused by **HYPOXIA**, requiring immediate ABC care, **NOT** drug therapy; therefore **ONLY** administer atropine in cases of bradycardia caused by vagal stimulation (e.g. suction).

Route: Intravenous/intra-osseous **administer as a rapid bolus**.

AGE	INITIAL DOSE	REPEAT DOSE	DOSE INTERVAL	VOLUME	MAXIMUM DOSE
≥12 years 600 micrograms per ml	600 micrograms*	600 micrograms*	3–5 minutes	1 ml	3 milligrams

Atropine   ATR

Route: Intravenous/intra-osseous **administer as a rapid bolus**.

AGE	INITIAL DOSE	REPEAT DOSE	DOSE INTERVAL	VOLUME	MAXIMUM DOSE
≥12 years 300 micrograms per ml	600 micrograms*	600 micrograms*	3–5 minutes	2 ml	3 milligrams

Route: Intravenous/intra-osseous **administer as a rapid bolus**.

AGE	INITIAL DOSE	REPEAT DOSE	DOSE INTERVAL	VOLUME	MAXIMUM DOSE
≥12 years 200 micrograms per ml	600 micrograms*	600 micrograms*	3–5 minutes	3 ml	3 milligrams

Route: Intravenous/intra-osseous **administer as a rapid bolus**.

AGE	INITIAL DOSE	REPEAT DOSE	DOSE INTERVAL	VOLUME	MAXIMUM DOSE
≥12 years 100 micrograms per ml	600 micrograms*	600 micrograms*	3–5 minutes	6 ml	3 milligrams

*The adult dosage can be given as 500 or 600 micrograms to a maximum of 3 milligrams depending on presentation available.

Benzylpenicillin (Penicillin G)   BPN

Presentation

Ampoule containing 600 milligrams of benzylpenicillin as powder.

Administered intravenously or intramuscularly.

NB Different concentrations and volumes of administration (refer to administration and dosage tables).

Indications

Suspected meningococcal disease in the presence of:

i) a non-blanching rash (the classical, haemorrhagic, non-blanching rash (may be petechial or purpuric) – seen in approximately 40% of infected children)

and

ii) signs/symptoms suggestive of meningococcal septicaemia (**refer to meningococcal meningitis and septicaemia guideline for signs/symptoms**).

Action

Antibiotic: broad-spectrum.

Contra-indications

Known severe penicillin allergy (more than a simple rash alone).

Additional Information

- Meningococcal septicaemia is commonest in children and young adults.
- It may be rapidly progressive and fatal.

Benzylpenicillin (Penicillin G)   BPN

● Early administration of benzylpenicillin improves outcome.

Dosage and Administration

Administer en route to hospital (unless already administered).

NB IV/IO and IM concentrations are different and have different
volumes of administration.

Route: Intravenous/Intra-osseous – by slow injection.

AGE	INITIAL DOSE	REPEAT DOSE	DOSE INTERVAL	VOLUME	MAXIMUM DOSE
Adult 1.2 grams dissolved in 19.2 ml of water for injection	1.2 grams	NONE	N/A	20 ml	1.2 grams

Route: Intramuscular (antero-lateral aspect of thigh or upper arm –
preferably in a well perfused area) if rapid intravascular access cannot be
obtained.

AGE	INITIAL DOSE	REPEAT DOSE	DOSE INTERVAL	VOLUME	MAXIMUM DOSE
Adult 1.2 grams dissolved in 3.2 ml of water for injection	1.2 grams	NONE	N/A	4 ml	1.2 grams

Chlorphenamine (Piriton)   CPH

Presentation

Ampoule containing 10 milligrams of chlorphenamine malleate in 1 ml.

Tablet containing 4 milligrams of chlorphenamine malleate.

Oral solution containing 2 milligrams of chlorphenamine malleate in 5 ml.

Indications

Severe anaphylactic reactions (when indicated, should follow initial treatment with IM adrenaline).

Symptomatic allergic reactions falling short of anaphylaxis but causing patient distress e.g. severe itching.

Actions

An antihistamine that blocks the effect of histamine released during a hypersensitivity (allergic) reaction.

Also has anticholinergic properties.

Contra-indications

Known hypersensitivity.

Children less than 1 year of age.

Cautions

Hypotension.

Epilepsy.

Glaucoma.

Chlorphenamine (Piriton)   CPH

Hepatic disease.

Prostatic disease.

Side Effects

Sedation.

Dry mouth.

Headache.

Blurred vision.

Psychomotor impairment.

Gastrointestinal disturbance.

Transient hypotension.

Convulsions (rare).

The elderly are more likely to suffer side effects.

Warn anyone receiving chlorphenamine against driving or undertaking any other complex psychomotor task, due to the sedative and psychomotor side effects.

Dosage and Administration

Route: Intravenous/intra-osseous – **SLOWLY** over 1 minute/intramuscular.

AGE	INITIAL DOSE	REPEAT DOSE	DOSE INTERVAL	VOLUME	MAXIMUM DOSE
Adult 10 milligrams in 1 ml	10 milligrams	NONE	N/A	1 ml	10 milligrams

Chlorphenamine (Piriton) CPH

Route: Oral (tablet).

AGE	INITIAL DOSE	REPEAT DOSE	DOSE INTERVAL	VOLUME	MAXIMUM DOSE
Adult 4 milligrams per tablet	4 milligrams	NONE	N/A	1 tablet	4 milligrams

Route: Oral (solution).

AGE	INITIAL DOSE	REPEAT DOSE	DOSE INTERVAL	VOLUME	MAXIMUM DOSE
Adult 2 milligrams in 5 ml	4 milligrams	NONE	N/A	10 ml	4 milligrams

Clopidogrel

Presentation

Tablet containing clopidogrel:

- 75 milligrams.
- 300 milligrams.

Indications

Acute ST segment elevation myocardial infarction (STEMI)

- In patients not already taking clopidogrel.
- Receiving thrombolytic treatment.
- Anticipated thrombolytic treatment.
- Anticipated primary percutaneous coronary intervention (PPCI).

Actions

Inhibits platelet aggregation.

Contra-indications

- Known allergy or sensitivity to clopidogrel.
- Severe liver impairment.
- Active pathological bleeding such as peptic ulcer or intracranial haemorrhage.
- Breastfeeding.

Cautions

As the likely benefits of a single dose of clopidogrel outweigh the potential risks, clopidogrel may be administered in:

- Pregnancy.

Clopidogrel

CLO

- Patients taking non-steroidal anti-inflammatory drugs (NSAIDs).
- Patients with renal impairment.

Side Effects

- Dyspepsia.
- Abdominal pain.
- Diarrhoea.
- Bleeding (gastrointestinal and intracranial) – the occurrence of severe bleeding is similar to that observed with the administration of aspirin.

Dosage and Administration

Adults aged 18–75 years with acute ST-elevation myocardial infarction (STEMI) receiving thrombolysis or anticipated primary PCI, as per locally agreed STEMI care pathways.

NOTE: To be administered in conjunction with aspirin unless there is a known aspirin allergy or sensitivity (refer to aspirin protocol for administration and dosage).

Route: Oral.

Clopidogrel

CLO

Patient care pathway: Thrombolysis.

AGE	INITIAL DOSE	REPEAT DOSE	DOSE INTERVAL	VOLUME	MAXIMUM DOSE
Adult 300 milligrams per tablet	300 milligrams	NONE	N/A	1 tablet	300 milligrams
Adult 75 milligrams per tablet	300 milligrams	NONE	N/A	4 tablets	300 milligrams

Patient care pathway: Primary percutaneous coronary intervention.

AGE	INITIAL DOSE	REPEAT DOSE	DOSE INTERVAL	VOLUME	MAXIMUM DOSE
Adult 300 milligrams per tablet	600 milligrams	NONE	N/A	2 tablets	600 milligrams
Adult 75 milligrams per tablet	600 milligrams	NONE	N/A	8 tablets	600 milligrams

Dexamethasone

Presentation

Ampoules of **intravenous** preparation 3.8 mg/ml.

Indications

Moderate/severe croup.

Actions

Corticosteroid – reduces subglottic inflammation.

Contra-indications

Previously diagnosed hypertension.

Systemic infection/sepsis.

Cautions

Upper airway compromise can be worsened by any procedure distressing the child – including the administration of medication and measuring blood pressure.

Side Effects

None.

Additional Information

Additional doses given acutely do not have additional benefits.

Dexamethasone

DEX

Dosage and Administration

Route: Oral.

> The intravenous preparation is administered ORALLY.

AGE	INITIAL DOSE	REPEAT DOSE	DOSE INTERVAL	VOLUME	MAXIMUM DOSE
11 years	N/A	N/A	N/A	N/A	N/A
10 years	N/A	N/A	N/A	N/A	N/A
9 years	N/A	N/A	N/A	N/A	N/A
8 years	N/A	N/A	N/A	N/A	N/A
7 years	N/A	N/A	N/A	N/A	N/A
6 years 3.8 milligrams per ml	3.8 milligrams	NONE	N/A	1 ml	3.8 milligrams
5 years 3.8 milligrams per ml	3.8 milligrams	NONE	N/A	1 ml	3.8 milligrams
4 years 3.8 milligrams per ml	3.8 milligrams	NONE	N/A	1 ml	3.8 milligrams
3 years 3.8 milligrams per ml	3.8 milligrams	NONE	N/A	1 ml	3.8 milligrams

Dexamethasone

DEX

Dosage and Administration

Route: Oral – *continued.*

AGE	INITIAL DOSE	REPEAT DOSE	DOSE INTERVAL	VOLUME	MAXIMUM DOSE
2 years 3.8 milligrams per ml	3.8 milligrams	NONE	N/A	1 ml	3.8 milligrams
18 months 3.8 milligrams per ml	3.8 milligrams	NONE	N/A	1 ml	3.8 milligrams
12 months 3.8 milligrams per ml	1.9 milligrams	NONE	N/A	0.5 ml	1.9 milligrams
9 months 3.8 milligrams per ml	1.9 milligrams	NONE	N/A	0.5 ml	1.9 milligrams
6 months 3.8 milligrams per ml	1.9 milligrams	NONE	N/A	0.5 ml	1.9 milligrams
3 months 3.8 milligrams per ml	1.9 milligrams	NONE	N/A	0.5 ml	1.9 milligrams
1 month 3.8 milligrams per ml	1.9 milligrams	NONE	N/A	0.5 ml	1.9 milligrams
Birth	N/A	N/A	N/A	N/A	N/A

Diazepam   DZP

Presentation

Ampoule containing 10 milligrams diazepam in an oil-in-water emulsion making up 2 ml.

Rectal tube containing 2.5 milligrams, 5 milligrams or 10 milligrams diazepam.

Indications

Fits longer than 5 minutes and **STILL FITTING**.

Repeated fits – not secondary to an uncorrected hypoxia or hypoglycaemic episode.

Status epilepticus.

Eclamptic fits (initiate treatment if fit lasts >2–3 minutes or if it is recurrent).

Symptomatic cocaine toxicity (severe hypertension, chest pain or fitting).

Actions

Central nervous system depressant, acts as an anticonvulsant and sedative.

Cautions

Respiratory depression.

Should be used with caution if alcohol, antidepressants or other CNS depressants have been taken as side effects are more likely.

Diazepam

DZP

Recent doses by carers/relatives should be taken into account when calculating the maximum cumulative dose.

Contra-indications

None.

Side Effects

Respiratory depression may occur, especially in the presence of alcohol, which enhances the depressive side effect of diazepam. In addition, opioid drugs also enhance the cardiac and respiratory depressive effect of diazepam.

Hypotension may occur. This may be significant if the patient has to be moved from a horizontal position to allow for extrication from an address. Caution should therefore be exercised and consideration given to either removing the patient flat or, if fitting has stopped and it is considered safe, allowing a 10 minute recovery period prior to removal.

Drowsiness and light-headedness, confusion and unsteadiness.

Occasionally amnesia may occur.

Additional Information

The intravenous route is preferred for terminating fits and thus, where IV access can be gained rapidly, this should be the first choice. Early consideration should be given to using the PR route when IV access cannot be rapidly and safely obtained, **which is particularly likely in the case of children**. In small children the PR route should be considered the first choice treatment and IV access sought subsequently.

Diazepam

DZP

NB If a **SINGLE** dose of diazepam has been administered via the PR route and IV access is subsequently available, a **SINGLE** dose of IV diazepam may be administered where required.

The earlier the drug is given the more likely the patient is to respond, which is why the rectal route is preferred in children, while the IV route is sought.

Diazepam should only be used if the patient has been fitting for >5 minutes (and is still fitting), or if fits recur in rapid succession without time for full recovery in between. There is no value in giving this drug 'preventatively' if the fit has ceased. **In any clearly sick or ill child, there must be no delay at the scene** while administering the drug, and if it is essential to give diazepam, this should be done en route to hospital.

Care must be taken when inserting the rectal tube and this should be inserted no more than 2.5 cm in children and 4–5 cm in adults. (All tubes have an insertion marker on nozzle.)

Dosage and Administration

Route: Intravenous/intra-osseous – administer **SLOWLY** titrated to response.

AGE	INITIAL DOSE	REPEAT DOSE	DOSE INTERVAL	VOLUME	MAXIMUM DOSE
Adult 10 milligrams in 2 ml	10 milligrams	10 milligrams	5 minutes	2 ml	20 milligrams

Diazepam

DZP

Route: Rectal (smaller dose).

AGE	INITIAL DOSE	REPEAT DOSE	DOSE INTERVAL	RECTAL TUBE	MAXIMUM DOSE
>12 years – Adult 10 milligrams in 2.5 ml	10 milligrams	NONE	N/A	1 × 10 milligram Tube	10 milligrams

NB If a **SINGLE** dose of diazepam has been given by the PR route and IV access is subsequently available, a **SINGLE** dose of IV diazepam may be given where required.

Route: Rectal (larger dose).

AGE	INITIAL DOSE	REPEAT DOSE	DOSE INTERVAL	RECTAL TUBE	MAXIMUM DOSE
>12 years – Adult 10 milligrams in 2.5 ml	20 milligrams	NONE	N/A	2 × 10 milligram Tube	20 milligrams

NB If a **SINGLE** dose of diazepam has been given by the PR route and IV access is subsequently available, a **SINGLE** dose of IV diazepam may be given where required.

Entonox

Presentation

Entonox is a combination of nitrous oxide 50% and oxygen 50%. It is stored in medical cylinders that have a blue body with white shoulders.

Indications

Moderate to severe pain.

Labour pains.

Actions

Inhaled analgesic agent.

Contra-indications

- Severe head injuries with impaired consciousness.
- Decompression sickness (the bends) where entonox can cause nitrogen bubbles within the blood stream to expand, aggravating the problem further. Consider anyone that has been diving within the previous 24 hours to be at risk.
- Violently disturbed psychiatric patients.

Cautions

Any patient at risk of having a pneumothorax, pneumomediastinum and/or a pneumoperitoneum e.g. polytrauma, penetrating torso injury.

Side Effects

Minimal side effects.

Entonox

Additional Information

Administration of entonox should be in conjunction with pain score monitoring.

Entonox's advantages include:

- Rapid analgesic effect with minimal side effects.
- No cardio-respiratory depression.
- Self-administered.
- Analgesic effect rapidly wears off.
- The 50% oxygen concentration is valuable in many medical and trauma conditions.
- Entonox can be administered whilst preparing to deliver other analgesics.

The usual precautions must be followed with regard to caring for the Entonox equipment and the cylinder MUST be inverted several times to mix the gases when temperatures are low.

Dosage and Administration

Adults:

- Entonox should be self-administered via a facemask or mouthpiece, after suitable instruction. It takes about **3–5 minutes** to be effective, but it may be **5–10 minutes** before maximum effect is achieved.

Children:

- Entonox is effective in children provided they are capable of following the administration instructions and can activate the demand valve.

Furosemide

Presentation

Ampoules containing furosemide 50 milligrams/5 ml.

Ampoules containing furosemide 40 milligrams/2 ml.

Pre-filled syringe containing furosemide 80 milligrams.

Indications

Pulmonary oedema secondary to left ventricular failure.

Actions

Furosemide is a potent diuretic with a rapid onset (within 30 minutes) and short duration.

Contra-indications

Pre-comatose state secondary to liver cirrhosis.

Severe renal failure with anuria.

Children under 18 years old.

Cautions

Hypokalaemia (low potassium) could induce arrhythmias.

Pregnancy.

Hypotensive patient.

Side Effects

Hypotension.

Gastro-intestinal disturbances.

Furosemide

FRM

Additional Information

Nitrates are the first-line treatment for acute pulmonary oedema. Use furosemide secondary to nitrates in the treatment of acute pulmonary oedema where transfer times to hospital are prolonged.

Dosage and Administration

Route: Intravenous – administer **SLOWLY OVER** 2 minutes.

AGE	INITIAL DOSE	REPEAT DOSE	DOSE INTERVAL	VOLUME	MAXIMUM DOSE
Adult 50 milligrams/ 5 ml	50 milligrams	NONE	N/A	5 ml	50 milligrams
Adult 20 milligrams/ 2 ml	40 milligrams	NONE	N/A	4 ml	40 milligrams
Adult 80 milligrams/ 8 ml (pre-filled syringe)	40 milligrams	NONE	N/A	4 ml	40 milligrams

Glucagon (Glucagen)

Presentation

Glucagon injection, 1 milligram of powder in vial for reconstitution with water for injection.

Indications

- Hypoglycaemia (blood glucose <4.0 millimoles per litre), especially in known diabetics.
- Clinically suspected hypoglycaemia where oral glucose administration is not possible.
- The unconscious patient, where hypoglycaemia is considered a likely cause.

Actions

Glucagon is a hormone that induces the conversion of glycogen to glucose in the liver, thereby raising blood glucose levels.

Contra-indications

- Low glycogen stores (e.g. recent use of glucagon).
- Hypoglycaemic seizures – glucose 10% IV is the preferred intervention.

Cautions

Avoid intramuscular administration of any drug when a patient is likely to require thrombolysis.

Glucagon (Glucagen)

Side Effects

- Nausea, vomiting.
- Diarrhoea.
- Acute hypersensitivity reaction (rare).
- Hypokalaemia.
- Hypotension.

Additional Information

- Glucagon should NOT be given by IV injection because of increased vomiting associated with IV use.

- Confirm effectiveness by checking blood glucose 5–10 minutes after administration (i.e. blood sugar >5.0 millimoles per litre).

- When treating hypoglycaemia, use all available clinical information to help decide between glucagon IM, oral glucose gel (40%), or glucose 10% IV (see advice below):

  - glucagon is relatively ineffective once body glycogen stores have been exhausted (especially hypoglycaemic, non-diabetic children). In such patients, use oral glucose gel smeared round the mouth or glucose 10% IV as first-line treatments

  - the newborn baby's liver has very limited glycogen stores, so hypoglycaemia may not be effectively treated using intramuscular glucagon (glucagon works by stimulating the liver to convert glycogen into glucose)

  - glucagon may also be ineffective in some instances of alcohol-induced hypoglycaemia

Glucagon (Glucagen) GLU

- consider oral glucose gel or glucose 10% IV as possible alternatives
- hypoglycaemic patients who fit should **preferably** be given glucose 10% IV.

Dosage and Administration

Route: Intramuscular – antero-lateral aspect of thigh or upper arm.

AGE	INITIAL DOSE	REPEAT DOSE	DOSE INTERVAL	VOLUME	MAXIMUM DOSE
Adult 1 milligram per vial	1 milligram	NONE	N/A	1 vial	1 milligram

NB If no response within 10 minutes, administer intravenous glucose – **refer to glucose 10% guideline**.

Glucose 10%   GLX

Presentation

500 ml pack of 10% glucose solution (50 grams).

Indications

Hypoglycaemia (blood glucose <4.0 millimoles per litre), especially in known diabetics.

Clinically suspected hypoglycaemia where oral glucose administration is not possible.

The unconscious patient, where hypoglycaemia is considered a likely cause.

Actions

Reversal of hypoglycaemia.

Cautions

Administer via a large gauge cannula into a large vein – a 10% concentration of glucose solution is an irritant to veins (especially in extravasation).

Additional Information

When treating hypoglycaemia, use all available clinical information to help decide between glucose 10% IV, glucose gel 40% oral gel, or glucagon IM.

Side Effects

None.

Glucose 10% **GLX**

Contra-indications

None.

Dosage and Administration

- If the patient has shown no response, the dose may be repeated after 5 minutes.

- If the patient has shown a **PARTIAL** response then a further infusion may be necessary, titrated to response to restore a normal GCS.

- If after the second dose there has been **NO** response, pre-alert and transport rapidly to further care. Consider an alternative diagnosis or the likelihood of a third dose en route benefitting the patient.

Route: Intravenous infusion.

AGE	INITIAL DOSE	REPEAT DOSE	DOSE INTERVAL	VOLUME	MAXIMUM DOSE
Adult 50 grams in 500 ml	10 grams	10 grams	5 minutes	100 ml	30 grams

Glucose 40% Oral Gel　　　GLG

Presentation

Plastic tube containing 25g glucose 40% oral gel.

Indications

Known or suspected hypoglycaemia in a conscious patient where there is no risk of choking or aspiration.

Actions

Rapid increase in blood glucose levels via buccal absorption.

Cautions

Altered consciousness – risk of choking or aspiration (in such circumstances glucose gel can be administered by soaking a gauze swab and placing it between the patient's lip and gum to aid absorption).

Side Effects

None.

Additional Information

Can be repeated as necessary in the hypoglycaemic patient.

Treatment failure should prompt the use of an alternative such as glucagon IM or glucose 10% IV.

(**Refer to glucagon guideline or glucose 10% guideline**).

Contra-indications

None.

Glucose 40% Oral Gel

GLG

Dosage and Administration

Route: Buccal – Measure blood glucose level after each dose.

AGE	INITIAL DOSE	REPEAT DOSE	DOSE INTERVAL	VOLUME	MAXIMUM DOSE*
Adult 10 grams in 25 grams of gel	10 grams	10 grams	5 minutes	1 tube	No limit

NB Assess more frequently in children who require a smaller dose for a response.

*Consider IM glucagon or IV glucose 10% if no clinical improvement.

Glyceryl Trinitrate (GTN, Suscard)

GTN

Presentation

Metered dose spray containing 400 micrograms glyceryl trinitrate per dose.

Tablets containing glyceryl trinitrate 2, 3 or 5 milligrams for buccal administration (depends on local ordering).

Indications

Cardiac chest pain due to angina or myocardial infarction.

Acute cardiogenic pulmonary oedema.

Actions

A potent vasodilator drug resulting in:

- Dilatation of coronary arteries/relief of coronary spasm.
- Dilatation of systemic veins resulting in lower pre-load.
- Reduced blood pressure.

Contra-indications

Hypotension (actual or estimated systolic blood pressure <90 mmHg).

Hypovolaemia.

Head trauma.

Cerebral haemorrhage.

Sildenafil (Viagra) and other related drugs – glyceryl trinitrate must not be given to patients who have taken sildenafil or related drugs within the previous 24 hours. Profound hypotension may occur.

Unconscious patients.

Glyceryl Trinitrate (GTN, Suscard)

GTN

Dosage and Administration

The oral mucosa must be moist for GTN absorption, moisten if necessary.

Route: Buccal/sub-lingual (spray under the patient's tongue and close mouth).

AGE	INITIAL DOSE	REPEAT DOSE	DOSE INTERVAL	TABLETS	MAXIMUM DOSE*
Adult 400 micrograms per dose spray	1–2 sprays	1–2 sprays	5–10 minutes	400–800 micrograms	No limit
Adult 2 milligrams per tablet	2 milligrams	2 milligrams	5–10 minutes	1 tablet	No limit
Adult 3 milligrams per tablet	3 milligrams	3 milligrams	5–10 minutes	1 tablet	No limit
Adult 5 milligrams per tablet	5 milligrams	5 milligrams	5–10 minutes	1 tablet	No limit

*The effect of the first dose should be assessed over 5 minutes; further doses can be administered provided the systolic blood pressure is >90 mmHg. Remove the tablet if side effects occur, for example, hypotension.

Heparin

Presentation

An ampoule of unfractionated heparin containing 5,000 units/ml.

Indications

ST Elevation Myocardial Infarction (STEMI) where heparin is required as adjunctive therapy with reteplase or tenecteplase to reduce the risk of re-infarction.

It is extremely important that the initial bolus dose is given at the earliest opportunity prior to administration of thrombolytic agents and a heparin infusion is commenced immediately on arrival at hospital.

A further intravenous bolus dose of 1,000 units heparin may be required if a heparin infusion **HAS NOT** commenced within 45 minutes of the original bolus of thrombolytic agent.

Recent trials have suggested that low molecular weight heparin may be useful in patients under 75 years of age (older patients have much higher bleeding risk with this treatment). Research is ongoing and local protocols should be followed.

Actions

Anticoagulant.

Side Effects

Haemorrhage – major or minor.

Heparin

Contra-indications

- **Haemophilia and other haemorrhagic disorders**.
- Thrombocytopenia.
- Recent cerebral haemorrhage.
- Severe hypertension.
- Severe liver disease.
- Oesophageal varices.
- Peptic ulcer.
- Major trauma.
- Recent surgery to eye or nervous system.
- Acute bacterial endocarditis.
- Spinal or epidural anaesthesia.

Additional Information

Analysis of MINAP data suggests inadequate anticoagulation following prehospital thrombolytic treatment is associated with increased risks of re-infarction.

AT HOSPITAL it is essential that the care of the patient is handed over as soon as possible to a member of hospital staff qualified to administer the second bolus (if not already given) and commence a heparin infusion.

Heparin

Dosage and Administration

Heparin dosage when administered with **RETEPLASE**.

Route: Intravenous single bolus unfractionated heparin.

AGE	INITIAL DOSE	REPEAT DOSE	DOSE INTERVAL	VOLUME	MAXIMUM DOSE
≥18	5,000 units	*See footnote	N/A	1 ml	5,000 units

Heparin dosage when administered with **TENECTEPLASE**.

Route: Intravenous single bolus unfractionated heparin.

AGE	WEIGHT	INITIAL DOSE	REPEAT DOSE	DOSE INTERVAL	VOLUME	MAXIMUM DOSE
≥18	<67 kg	4,000 units	*See footnote	N/A	0.8 ml	4,000 units
≥18	≥67 kg	5,000 units	*See footnote	N/A	1 ml	5,000 units

*A further intravenous bolus dose of 1,000 units heparin may be required if a heparin infusion **HAS NOT** commenced within 45 minutes of the original bolus of thrombolytic agent.

Hydrocortisone

HYC

Presentation

An ampoule containing 100 milligrams hydrocortisone as either sodium succinate or sodium phosphate in 1 ml.

An ampoule containing 100 milligrams hydrocortisone sodium succinate for reconstitution with up to 2 ml of water.

Indications

Severe or life-threatening asthma.

Anaphylaxis.

Adrenal crisis (including Addisonian crisis) – sudden severe deficiency of steroids (occurs in patients on long-term steroid therapy for whatever reason) producing circulatory collapse with or without hypoglycaemia. Administer hydrocortisone to:

1. Patients in an established adrenal crisis.
2. Steroid-dependent patients who have become unwell to prevent them having an adrenal crisis – if in doubt, it is better to administer hydrocortisone.

Actions

Glucocorticoid drug that reduces inflammation and suppresses the immune response.

Contra-indications

Known allergy (which will be to the sodium succinate or sodium phosphate rather than the hydrocortisone itself).

Hydrocortisone   **HYC**

Cautions

None relevant to a single dose.

Avoid intramuscular administration if patient likely to require thrombolysis.

Side Effects

Sodium phosphate may cause burning or itching sensation in the groin if administered too quickly.

Dosage and Administration

1. **Asthma and adrenal crisis**. NB If there is any doubt about previous steroid administration, it is better to administer hydrocortisone.

Route: Intravenous (**SLOW** injection over a minimum of 2 minutes to avoid side effects)/intra-osseous OR intramuscular (when IV access is impossible).

AGE	INITIAL DOSE	REPEAT DOSE	DOSE INTERVAL	VOLUME	MAXIMUM DOSE
Adult 100 milligrams in 1 ml	100 milligrams	NONE	N/A	1 ml	100 milligrams

Hydrocortisone

HYC

Route: Intravenous (**SLOW** injection over a minimum of 2 minutes to avoid side effects)/intra-osseous OR intramuscular (when IV access is impossible).

AGE	INITIAL DOSE	REPEAT DOSE	DOSE INTERVAL	VOLUME	MAXIMUM DOSE
Adult 100 milligrams in 2 ml	100 milligrams	NONE	N/A	2 ml	100 milligrams

2. Anaphylaxis

Route: Intravenous (**SLOW** injection over a minimum of 2 minutes to avoid side effects)/intra-osseous OR intramuscular (when IV access is impossible).

AGE	INITIAL DOSE	REPEAT DOSE	DOSE INTERVAL	VOLUME	MAXIMUM DOSE
Adult 100 milligrams in 1 ml	200 milligrams	NONE	N/A	2 ml	200 milligrams

Route: Intravenous (**SLOW** injection over a minimum of 2 minutes to avoid side effects)/intra-osseous OR intramuscular (when IV access is impossible).

AGE	INITIAL DOSE	REPEAT DOSE	DOSE INTERVAL	VOLUME	MAXIMUM DOSE
Adult 100 milligrams in 2 ml	200 milligrams	NONE	N/A	4 ml	200 milligrams

Ibuprofen

Presentation

Solution or suspension containing ibuprofen 100 milligrams in 5 ml.

Tablet containing 200 milligrams or 400 milligrams.

Indications

Relief of mild to moderate pain and/or high temperature.

Soft tissue injuries.

Best when used as part of a balanced analgesic regimen.

Actions

Analgesic (relieves pain).

Antipyretic (reduces temperature).

Anti-inflammatory (reduces inflammation).

Contra-indications

Do **NOT** administer if the patient is:

- Dehydrated.
- Hypovolaemic.
- Known to have renal insufficiency.
- Suffering active upper gastrointestinal disturbance
  e.g. oesophagitis, peptic ulcer, dyspepsia.
- Pregnant.

Ibuprofen

Avoid giving further non-steroidal anti-inflammatory drugs (NSAIDs) i.e. ibuprofen, if an NSAID containing product (e.g. Diclofenac, Naproxen) has been used within the previous four hours or if the maximum cumulative daily dose has already been given.

Cautions

Asthma: Use cautiously in asthmatic patients due to the possible risk of hypersensitivity and bronchoconstriction. If an asthmatic has not used NSAIDs previously, do not use acutely in the prehospital setting.

Elderly: Exercise caution in older patients (>65 years old) that have not used and tolerated NSAIDs recently.

Side Effects

May cause nausea, vomiting and tinnitus.

Dosage and Administration

Route: Oral.

AGE	INITIAL DOSE	REPEAT DOSE	DOSE INTERVAL	VOLUME	MAXIMUM DOSE
12 years – adult	400 milligrams	400 milligrams	8 hours	Varies	1.2 grams per 24 hours

NB

- Combinations of both paracetamol and ibuprofen should not be given together. Only consider alternating these agents if the distress persists or recurs before the next dose is due.
- Given up to 3 times a day, preferably following food.

Ipratropium Bromide (Atrovent)

Presentation

Nebules containing ipratropium bromide 250 micrograms in 1 ml or 500 micrograms in 2 ml.

Indications

Acute severe or life-threatening asthma.

Acute asthma unresponsive to salbutamol.

Exacerbation of chronic obstructive pulmonary disease (COPD), unresponsive to salbutamol.

Actions

1. Ipratropium bromide is an antimuscarinic bronchodilator drug. It may provide short-term relief in acute asthma, but beta2 agonists (such as salbutamol) generally work more quickly.

2. Ipratropium is considered of greater benefit in:
   a. children suffering acute asthma
   b. adults suffering with COPD.

Contra-Indications

None in the emergency situation.

Cautions

Ipratropium should be used with care in patients with:

- Glaucoma (protect the eyes from mist).

Ipratropium Bromide (Atrovent)   IPR

- Pregnancy and breastfeeding.
- Prostatic hyperplasia.

If COPD is a possibility limit nebulisation to six minutes.

Side Effects

Headache.

Nausea and vomiting.

Dry mouth (common).

Difficulty in passing urine and/or constipation.

Tachycardia/arrhythmia.

Paroxysmal tightness of the chest.

Allergic reaction.

Dosage and Administration

- **In life-threatening or acute severe asthma:** undertake a **TIME CRITICAL** transfer to the **NEAREST SUITABLE RECEIVING HOSPITAL** and provide nebulisation en route.
- If COPD is a possibility limit nebulisation to six minutes.

Route: Nebuliser with 6–8 litres per minute oxygen (**refer to oxygen guideline**).

Ipratropium Bromide (Atrovent)

IPR

Route: Nebuliser with 6–8 litres per minute oxygen (**refer to oxygen guideline**).

AGE	INITIAL DOSE	REPEAT DOSE	DOSE INTERVAL	VOLUME	MAXIMUM DOSE
Adult 250 micrograms in 1 ml	500 micrograms	NONE	N/A	2 ml	500 micrograms

Route: Nebuliser with 6–8 litres per minute oxygen (**refer to oxygen guideline**).

AGE	INITIAL DOSE	REPEAT DOSE	DOSE INTERVAL	VOLUME	MAXIMUM DOSE
Adult 500 micrograms in 2 ml	500 micrograms	NONE	N/A	2 ml	500 micrograms

Metoclopramide (Maxolon)   MTC

Presentation

Ampoule containing metoclopramide 10 milligrams in 2 ml.

Indications

The treatment of nausea or vomiting in adults aged 20 and over.

Prevention and treatment of nausea and vomiting following administration of morphine sulphate.

Actions

An anti-emetic which acts centrally as well as on the gastrointestinal tract.

Contra-indications

- Age less than 20 years.
- Renal failure.
- Phaeochromocytoma.
- Gastrointestinal obstruction.
- Perforation/haemorrhage/3–4 days after GI surgery.

Cautions

If patient is likely to require thrombolysis then intramuscular administration of any drug should be avoided.

Avoid in cases of drug overdose.

Metoclopramide (Maxolon)　　MTC

Side Effects

Severe extra-pyramidal effects are more common in children and young adults.

- Drowsiness and restlessness.
- Cardiac conduction abnormalities following IV administration.
- Diarrhoea.
- Rash.

Additional Information

Metoclopramide should always be given in a separate syringe to morphine sulphate. The drugs must not be mixed.

Dosage and Administration

Route: Intravenous – administer over 2 minutes.

AGE	INITIAL DOSE	REPEAT DOSE	DOSE INTERVAL	VOLUME	MAXIMUM DOSE
Adult 10 milligrams in 2 ml	10 milligrams	NONE	N/A	2 ml	10 milligrams

NB Monitor pulse, blood pressure, respiratory rate and cardiac rhythm before, during and after administration.

Patient's Own Buccal Midazolam for Convulsions

Presentation

Presented in a glass bottle containing 5 ml of midazolam, 10 milligrams per 1 ml and supplied with four 1 ml syringes to draw up the dose.

Indications

Buccal Midazolam can be used as an anticonvulsant for generalised **convulsions** lasting **more than 5 minutes**, as they may not stop spontaneously.

Ambulance paramedics and technicians can administer the patient's own prescribed midazolam provided they are competent to administer buccal medication and are familiar with midazolam's indications, actions and side effects. Those that are not familiar with the use of this medication should use rectal (PR) or intravenous (IV) diazepam instead.

NB If the child continues fitting **10 minutes after their first dose of anticonvulsant**, they should receive intravenous **diazepam** for any further anticonvulsant treatment. If it is not possible to gain vascular access for the second dose of medication, no further drug treatment should be used, even if this means that the child continues to fit i.e. do not give a second dose of buccal or rectal medication.

Where a generalised convulsion continues ten minutes after the second anticonvulsant, senior medical advice should be sought.

Contra-indications

None.

Patient's Own Buccal Midazolam for Convulsions

MDZ

Actions

Midazolam has a sedative action similar to that of diazepam but of shorter duration. The onset of action usually occurs within five minutes, but is dependent on the route of administration. In 80% of episodes convulsions have stopped after ten minutes.

Side Effects

The side effects of buccal midazolam are similar in effect to IV administration, although, the timings may differ:

- Respiratory depression.
- Hypotension.
- Drowsiness.
- Muscle weakness.
- Slurred speech.
- Occasionally agitation, restlessness and disorientation may occur.

Additional Information

- **Midazolam is a benzodiazepine drug, which is now being administered by carers to treat convulsions as an alternative to rectal diazepam.**
- Some patients may have a Patient Specific Direction (PSD) drawn up by their specialist, customised to the specific nature of their convulsions. This is especially true of patients with learning disabilities living in residential care homes. Whenever possible check with the carers for the existence of a PSD for the patient, as this will normally give further guidance on treatment and when the patient should be further

assessed.

Patient's Own Buccal Midazolam for Convulsions

MDZ

The above guidance only applies to the administration of the patient's own supply of midazolam.

Dosage and Administration

Route: buccal (administered by carers).

Dosage – individual tailored dose as per the patient's individualised treatment plan.

Administration

The required dose is drawn up and half the dose is administered quickly to each side of the lower buccal cavity (between the cheek and gum).

NB If a generalised convulsion continues ten minutes after the second dose, senior medical advice should be sought.

Misoprostol

Presentation

Tablet containing misoprostol:

- 200 micrograms.

Indications

Postpartum haemorrhage within 24 hours of delivery of the infant where bleeding from the uterus is uncontrollable by uterine massage.

Miscarriage with life-threatening bleeding and a confirmed diagnosis e.g. where a patient has gone home with medical management and starts to bleed.

Both syntometrine and ergometrine are contra-indicated in hypertension (BP >140/90); in this case misoprostol (or preferably syntocinon if available) should be administered instead.

In all other circumstances misoprostol should only be used if syntometrine or other oxytocics are unavailable or if they have been ineffective at reducing haemorrhage after 15 mins.

Actions

Stimulates contraction of the uterus.

Onset of action 7–10 minutes.

Contra-indications

- Known hypersensitivity to misoprostol.
- Active labour.
- Possible multiple pregnancy/known or suspected fetus in utero.

Misoprostol

Side Effects

- Abdominal pain.
- Nausea and vomiting.
- Diarrhoea.
- Pyrexia.
- Shivering.

Additional Information

Syntometrine and misoprostol reduce bleeding from a pregnant uterus through different pathways; therefore if one drug has not been effective after 15 mins, the other may be administered in addition.

Dosage and Administration

- Administer orally unless the patient is unable to swallow.
- The vaginal route is not appropriate in postpartum haemorrhage.

Route: Oral.

AGE	INITIAL DOSE	REPEAT DOSE	DOSE INTERVAL	VOLUME	MAXIMUM DOSE
Adult 200 micrograms per tablet	600 micrograms	NONE	N/A	3 tablets	600 micrograms

Misoprostol

Route: Rectal.

NB At the time of publication there is no rectal preparation of misoprostol – therefore the same tablets can be administered orally or rectally.

AGE	INITIAL DOSE	REPEAT DOSE	DOSE INTERVAL	VOLUME	MAXIMUM DOSE
Adult 200 micrograms per tablet	1 mg	NONE	N/A	5 tablets	1 mg

Morphine Sulphate

MOR

Presentation

Parenteral — ampoules containing morphine sulphate 10 milligrams in 1 ml.

Oral — vials containing morphine sulphate 10 milligrams in 5 ml.

Indications

Pain associated with suspected myocardial infarction (analgesic of first choice).

Severe pain as a component of a balanced analgesia regimen.

The decision about which analgesia and which route should be guided by clinical judgement.

Actions

Morphine is a strong opioid analgesic. It is particularly useful for treating continuous, severe musculoskeletal and soft tissue pain.

Morphine produces sedation, euphoria and analgesia; it may both depress respiration and induce hypotension.

Histamine is released following morphine administration and this may contribute to its vasodilatory effects. This may also account for the urticaria and bronchoconstriction that are sometimes seen.

Contra-indications

Do **NOT** administer morphine in the following circumstances:

● Children under 1 year of age.

Morphine Sulphate

MOR

- Respiratory depression (adult <10 breaths per minute, child <20 breaths per minute).
- Hypotension (actual, not estimated, systolic blood pressure <90 mmHg in adults, <80 mmHg in school children, <70 mmHg in pre-school children).
- Head injury with significantly impaired level of consciousness (e.g. below P on the AVPU scale or below 9 on the GCS).
- Known hypersensitivity to morphine.
- Extreme headache.

Cautions

Known severe renal or hepatic impairment – smaller doses may be used carefully and titrated to effect.

Use with **extreme** caution (minimal doses) during pregnancy. **NOTE:** Not to be used for labour pain where entonox is the analgesic of choice.

Use morphine **WITH GREAT CAUTION** in patients with chest injuries, particularly those with any respiratory difficulty, although if respiration is inhibited by pain, analgesia may actually improve respiratory status.

Any patients with other respiratory problems e.g. asthma, COPD.

Head injury. Agitation following head injury may be due to acute brain injury, hypoxia or pain. The decision to administer analgesia to an agitated head injured patient is a clinical one. It is vital that if such a patient receives opioids they are closely monitored since opioids can cause disproportionate respiratory depression, which may ultimately lead to an elevated intracranial pressure through a raised arterial pCO_2.

Morphine Sulphate   MOR

Acute alcohol intoxication. All opioid drugs potentiate the central nervous system depressant effects of alcohol and they should therefore be used with great caution in patients who have consumed significant quantities of alcohol.

Medications. Prescribed antidepressants, sedatives or major tranquillisers may potentiate the respiratory and cardiovascular depressant effects of morphine.

Side Effects

- Respiratory depression.
- Cardiovascular depression.
- Nausea and vomiting.
- Drowsiness.
- Pupillary constriction.

Additional Information

Morphine is a Class A controlled drug under Schedule 2 of the Misuse of Drugs Regulations 1985, and must be stored and its prescription and administration documented in accordance with these regulations.

Morphine is not licensed for use in children but its use has been approved by the Medicines and Healthcare products Regulatory Agency (MHRA) for 'off label' use. This means that it can legally be administered under these guidelines by paramedics.

Unused morphine in open vials or syringes must be discarded in the presence of a witness.

Morphine Sulphate MOR

Special Precautions

Naloxone can be used to reverse morphine related respiratory or cardiovascular depression. It should be carefully titrated after assessment and appropriate management of ABC for that particular patient and situation (**refer to naloxone guideline**).

Morphine frequently induces nausea or vomiting which may be potentiated by the movement of the ambulance. Titrating to the lowest dose to achieve analgesia will reduce the risk of vomiting. The use of an anti-emetics should also be considered whenever administering any opioid analgesic (**refer to ondansetron and metoclopramide guidelines**).

Dosage and Administration

Administration must be in conjunction with pain score monitoring (**refer to pain assessment guidelines**).

Intravenous morphine takes a minimum of 2–3 minutes before starting to take effect, reaching its peak between 10–20 minutes.

The absorption of intramuscular, subcutaneous or oral morphine is variable particularly in patients with major trauma, shock and cardiac conditions; these routes should preferably be avoided if the circumstances favour intravenous or intra-osseous administration.

Morphine **should be** diluted with sodium chloride 0.9% to make a concentration of 10 milligrams in 10 ml (1 milligram in 1 ml) unless it is being administered by the intramuscular or subcutaneous route when it should not be diluted.

Morphine Sulphate **MOR**

ADULTS – If pain is not reduced to a tolerable level after 10 milligrams of IV/IO morphine, then further **2 milligram** doses may be administered by slow IV/IO injection every 5 minutes to **20 milligrams maximum**. The patient should be closely observed throughout the remaining treatment and transfer. Care should be taken with elderly patients who may be more susceptible to complications and in whom smaller doses of morphine may be adequate.

CHILDREN – The doses and volumes given below are for the initial and maximum doses. Administer **0.1 ml/kg** (equal to **0.1 milligrams/kg**) as an initial slow IV injection over 2 minutes. If pain is not reduced to a tolerable level after 5 minutes then a further dose of up to **0.1 milligrams/kg**, titrated to response, may be repeated (**maximum dose 0.2 milligrams/kg**).

NOTE: Peak effect of each dose may not occur until 10–20 minutes after administration.

Route: Intravenous/intra-osseous – administer by slow IV injection (rate of approximately 2 milligram per minute up to appropriate dose for age). Observe the patient for at least 5 minutes after completion of initial dose before repeating the dose if required.

AGE	INITIAL DOSE	REPEAT DOSE	DOSE INTERVAL	DILUTED CONCENTRATION	VOL	MAX DOSE
Adult	10 milligrams	10 milligrams	5 minutes	10 milligrams in 10 ml	10 ml	20 milligrams

Morphine Sulphate

Route: Oral.

AGE	INITIAL DOSE	REPEAT DOSE	DOSE INTERVAL	DILUTED CONCENTRATION	VOL	MAX DOSE
Adult	20 milligrams	20 milligrams	60 minutes	10 milligrams in 5 ml	10 ml	40 milligrams

NB Only administer via the oral route in patients with major trauma, shock or cardiac conditions if the IV/IO routes are not accessible.

Route: Intramuscular/subcutaneous.

AGE	INITIAL DOSE	REPEAT DOSE	DOSE INTERVAL	DILUTED CONCENTRATION	VOL	MAX DOSE
Adult	10 milligrams	10 milligrams	60 minutes	10 milligrams in 1 ml	1 ml	20 milligrams

NB Only administer via the intramuscular or subcutaneous route in patients with major trauma, shock or cardiac conditions if the IV/IO routes are not accessible.

Naloxone Hydrochloride (Narcan)

NLX

Presentation

Naloxone hydrochloride 400 micrograms per 1 ml ampoule.

Indications

Opioid overdose producing respiratory, cardiovascular and central nervous system depression.

Overdose of either an opioid analgesic, e.g. dextropropoxyphene, codeine, or a compound analgesic e.g. co-codamol (combination of codeine and paracetamol).

Unconsciousness, associated with respiratory depression of unknown cause, where opioid overdose is a possibility.

Reversal of respiratory and central nervous system depression in a neonate following maternal opioid use during labour.

Actions

Antagonism of the effects (including respiratory depression) of opioid drugs.

Contra-indications

Neonates born to opioid addicted mothers – produces serious withdrawal effects. Emphasis should be on bag-valve-mask ventilation and oxygenation – as with all patients.

Naloxone Hydrochloride (Narcan)   **NLX**

Side Effects

In patients who are physically dependent on opiates, naloxone may precipitate violent withdrawal symptoms, including cardiac arrhythmias. It is better, in these cases, to titrate the dose of naloxone as described to effectively reverse the cardiac and respiratory depression, but still leave the patient in a 'groggy' state with regular re-assessment of ventilation and circulation.

Additional information

When indicated, naloxone should be administered via the intravenous route.

If IV access is impossible, naloxone may be administered intramuscularly, **undiluted** (into the outer aspect of the thigh or upper arm), but absorption may be unpredictable.

Opioid induced respiratory and cardiovascular depression can be fatal.

When used, naloxone's effects are **short lived** and once its effects have worn off respiratory and cardiovascular depression can recur with fatal consequences. **All** cases of opioid overdose should be transported to hospital, even if the initial response to naloxone has been good. If the patient refuses hospitalisation, consider, if the patient consents, a loading dose of **800 micrograms IM** to minimise the risk described above.

Naloxone Hydrochloride (Narcan)   NLX

Dosage and Administration

Respiratory arrest/extreme respiratory depression.

- If there is no response after the initial dose, repeat every 3 minutes, up to the maximum dose, until an effect is noted. **NB** The half-life of naloxone is short.

- Known or potentially aggressive adults suffering respiratory depression: Dilute up to 800 micrograms (2 ml) of naloxone into 8 ml of water for injections or sodium chloride 0.9% to a total volume of 10 ml and administer **SLOWLY**, titrating to response, 1 ml at a time.

Route: Intravenous/intra-osseous – administer **SLOWLY** 1 ml at a time. Titrated to response relieving respiratory depression but maintain patient in 'groggy' state.

AGE	INITIAL DOSE	REPEAT DOSE	DOSE INTERVAL	VOLUME	MAXIMUM DOSE
12 years – adult 400 micrograms in 1 ml	400 micrograms	400 micrograms	3 minutes	1 ml	4400 micrograms

Naloxone Hydrochloride (Narcan)

Respiratory arrest/extreme respiratory depression where the IV/IO route is unavailable or the ambulance clinician is not trained to administer drugs via the IV/IO route.

- If there is no response after the initial dose, repeat every 3 minutes, up to the maximum dose, until an effect is noted. **NB** The half-life of naloxone is short.

- **For adults when administering naloxone via the intramuscular route:** Administering large volumes intramuscularly could lead to poor absorption and/or tissue damage; therefore divide the dose where necessary and practicable. Vary the site of injection for repeated doses; appropriate sites include: buttock (gluteus maximus), thigh (vastus lateralis), lateral hip (gluteus medius) and upper arm (deltoid).

Route: Intramuscular – initial dose.

AGE	INITIAL DOSE	REPEAT DOSE	DOSE INTERVAL	VOLUME	MAXIMUM DOSE
12 years – adult 400 micrograms in 1 ml	400 micrograms	See page 137	3 minutes	1 ml	4400 micrograms

Naloxone Hydrochloride (Narcan)   **NLX**

Route: Intramuscular – repeat dose.

AGE	INITIAL DOSE	REPEAT DOSE	DOSE INTERVAL	VOLUME	MAXIMUM DOSE
12 years – adult 400 micrograms in 1 ml	See page 136	400 micrograms	3 minutes	1 ml	4400 micrograms

Reversal of respiratory and central nervous system depression in a neonate following maternal opioid use during labour.

● Administer a single dose only.

Route: Intramuscular.

AGE	INITIAL DOSE	REPEAT DOSE	DOSE INTERVAL	VOLUME	MAXIMUM DOSE
Birth 400 micrograms in 1 ml	200 micrograms	NONE	N/A	0.5 ml	200 micrograms

Ondansetron

Presentation

Ampoule containing 4 milligrams of ondansetron (as hydrochloride) in 2 ml.

Ampoule containing 8 milligrams of ondansetron (as hydrochloride) in 4 ml.

NB Both these preparations share the same concentration (2 milligrams in 1 ml).

Indications

Adults:

- Prevention and treatment of opiate-induced nausea and vomiting e.g. morphine sulphate.
- Treatment of nausea or vomiting.

Children:

- Prevention and treatment of opiate-induced nausea and vomiting e.g. morphine sulphate.
- For travel associated nausea or vomiting.

Actions

An anti-emetic that blocks 5HT receptors both centrally and in the gastrointestinal tract.

Contra-indications

Known sensitivity to ondansetron.

Infants <1 month old.

Ondansetron

Cautions

QT interval prolongation (avoid concomitant administration of drugs that prolong QT interval).

Hepatic impairment.

Pregnancy.

Breastfeeding.

Side Effects

- Hiccups.
- Constipation.
- Flushing.
- Hypotension.
- Chest pain.
- Arrhythmias.
- Bradycardia.
- Headache.
- Seizures.
- Movement disorders.
- Injection site reactions.

Additional Information

Ondansetron should always be given in a separate syringe to morphine sulphate – the drugs must **NOT** be mixed.

Ondansetron should **NOT** be routinely administered in the management of childhood gastroenteritis.

Ondansetron

ODT

Dosage and Administration

Note: Two preparations exist (4 mg in 2 ml and 8 mg in 4 ml). They share the same concentration i.e. 2 milligrams in 1 ml.

Route: Intravenous (**SLOW** IV injection over 2 minutes) /intramuscular.

AGE	INITIAL DOSE	REPEAT DOSE	DOSE INTERVAL	VOLUME	MAXIMUM DOSE
12 years – adult 2 milligrams in 1 ml	4 milligrams	NONE	N/A	2 ml	4 milligrams

NB Monitor pulse, blood pressure, respiratory rate and cardiac rhythm before, during and after administration.

Oxygen

Presentation

Oxygen (O_2) is a gas provided in compressed form in a cylinder. It is also available in liquid form, in a system adapted for ambulance use. It is fed via a regulator and flow meter to the patient by means of plastic tubing and an oxygen mask/nasal cannulae.

Indications

Children

● Significant illness and/or injury.

Adults

● Critical illnesses requiring high levels of supplemental oxygen (refer to page 150).

● Serious illnesses requiring moderate levels of supplemental oxygen if the patient is hypoxaemic (refer to page 151).

● COPD and other conditions requiring controlled or low-dose oxygen therapy (refer to page 152).

● Conditions for which patients should be monitored closely but oxygen therapy is not required unless the patient is hypoxaemic (refer to page 153).

Actions

Essential for cell metabolism. Adequate tissue oxygenation is essential for normal physiological function.

Oxygen assists in reversing hypoxia, by raising the concentration of inspired oxygen. Hypoxia will, however, only improve if respiratory effort or ventilation and tissue perfusion are adequate.

Oxygen

If ventilation is inadequate or absent, assisting or completely taking over the patient's ventilation is essential to reverse hypoxia.

Contra-indications

Explosive environments.

Cautions

Oxygen increases the fire hazard at the scene of an incident.

Defibrillation – ensure pads firmly applied to reduce spark hazard.

Side Effects

Non-humidified O_2 is drying and irritating to mucous membranes over a period of time.

In patients with COPD there is a risk that even moderately high doses of inspired oxygen can produce increased carbon dioxide levels which may cause respiratory depression and this may lead to respiratory arrest. Refer to page **147** for guidance.

Dosage and Administration

- Measure oxygen saturation (SpO_2) in all patients using pulse oximetry.
- For the administration of **moderate** levels of supplemented oxygen nasal cannulae are recommended in preference to simple face mask as they offer more flexible dose range.
- Patients with tracheostomy or previous laryngectomy may require alternative appliances e.g. tracheostomy masks.
- Entonox may be administered when required.
- Document oxygen administration.

Oxygen

Children

● **ALL** children with significant illness and/or injury should receive **HIGH** levels of supplementary oxygen.

Adults

● Administer the initial oxygen dose until a reliable oxygen saturation reading is obtained.

● If the desired oxygen saturation cannot be maintained with simple face mask change to reservoir mask (non-rebreathe mask).

● For dosage and administration of supplemental oxygen refer to pages **144–147**.

● For conditions where **NO** supplemental oxygen is required unless the patient is hypoxaemic refer to page **148**.

Oxygen

High levels of supplemental oxygen for adults with critical illnesses

Target saturation 94–98% Administer the initial oxygen dose until the vital signs are normal, then reduce oxygen dose and aim for target saturation within the range of **94–98%** as per the table below.

Condition	Initial dose	Method of administration
• Cardiac arrest or resuscitation: – basic life support – advanced life support – foreign body airway obstruction – traumatic cardiac arrest – maternal resuscitation. • Carbon monoxide poisoning.	Maximum dose until the vital signs are normal NOTE – **Some oxygen saturation monitors cannot differentiate between carboxyhaemoglobin and oxyhaemoglobin owing to carbon monoxide poisoning**	Bag-valve-mask
• Major trauma: – abdominal trauma – burns and scalds – electrocution – head trauma – limb trauma – neck and back trauma (spinal) – pelvic trauma – the immersion incident – thoracic trauma – trauma in pregnancy.	15 litres per minute	Reservoir mask (non-rebreathe mask)

Oxygen

OXG

High levels of supplemental oxygen for adults with critical illnesses

Target saturation 94–98%

Administer the initial oxygen dose until the vital signs are normal, then reduce oxygen dose and aim for target saturation within the range of **94–98%** as per the table below.

Condition	Initial dose	Method of administration
• Anaphylaxis • Major pulmonary haemorrhage • Sepsis e.g. meningococcal septicaemia • Shock	15 litres per minute	Reservoir mask (non-rebreathe mask)
• Active convulsion • Hypothermia	Administer 15 litres per minute until a reliable SpO₂ measurement can be obtained and then adjust oxygen flow to aim for target saturation within the range of **94–98%**	Reservoir mask (non-rebreathe mask)

Oxygen

OXG

Moderate levels of supplemental oxygen for adults with serious illnesses if the patient is hypoxaemic

Target saturation 94–98%	Administer the initial oxygen dose until a reliable SpO_2 measurement is available, then adjust oxygen flow to aim for target saturation within the range of **94–98%** as per the table below.		
Condition		**Initial dose**	**Method of administration**
• Acute hypoxaemia (cause not yet diagnosed) • Deterioration of lung fibrosis or other interstitial lung disease • Acute asthma		**SpO_2 <85%** 10–15 litres per minute	Reservoir mask (non-rebreathe mask)
• Acute heart failure • Pneumonia • Lung cancer • Postoperative breathlessness		**SpO_2 ≥85–93%** 2–6 litres per minute	Nasal cannulae
• Pulmonary embolism • Pleural effusions • Pneumothorax • Severe anaemia • Sickle cell crisis		**SpO_2 ≥85–93%** 5–10 litres per minute	Simple face mask

Oxygen

OXG

Controlled or low-dose supplemental oxygen for adults with COPD and other conditions requiring controlled or low-dose oxygen therapy

Target saturation 88–92%

Administer the initial oxygen dose until a reliable SpO_2 measurement is available, then adjust oxygen flow to aim for target saturation within the range of **88–92%** or **prespecified range** detailed on the patient's alert card, as per the table below.

Condition	Initial dose	Method of administration
• Chronic obstructive pulmonary disease (COPD)	4 litres per minute	28% Venturi mask or patient's own mask
• Exacerbation of cystic fibrosis		**NB** If respiratory rate is >30 breaths/min using Venturi mask set flow rate to 50% above the minimum
• Chronic neuromuscular disorders	4 litres per minute	28% Venturi mask or patient's own mask
• Chest wall disorders		
• Morbid obesity (body mass index >40 kg/m²)		
	5–10 litres per minute	Simple face mask

NB If the oxygen saturation remains below 88% change to simple face mask.

NB Critical illness **AND** COPD/or other risk factors for hypercapnia.

If a patient with COPD or other risk factors for hypercapnia sustains or develops critical illness/injury ensure the same target saturations as indicated in HIGH levels page **144–145**.

Oxygen

No supplemental oxygen required for adults with these conditions unless the patient is hypoxaemic but patients should be monitored closely

Target saturation 94–98%

If hypoxaemic (SpO$_2$ <94%) administer the initial oxygen dose, then adjust oxygen flow to aim for target saturation within the range of **94–98%**, as per the table below.

Condition	Initial dose	Method of administration
• Myocardial infarction and acute coronary syndromes • Stroke • Cardiac rhythm disturbance • Non-traumatic chest pain/discomfort • Implantable cardioverter defibrillator firing	**SpO$_2$ <85%** 10–15 litres per minute	Reservoir mask (non-rebreathe mask)
	SpO$_2$ ≥85–93% 2–6 litres per minute	Nasal cannulae

• Pregnancy and obstetric emergencies:
  – birth imminent
  – haemorrhage during pregnancy
  – pregnancy induced hypertension
  – vaginal bleeding.
• Abdominal pain
• Headache
• Hyperventilation syndrome or dysfunctional breathing
	SpO$_2$ ≥85–93%
	5–10 litres per minute
		Simple face mask

Oxygen

OXG

No supplemental oxygen required for adults with these conditions unless the patient is hypoxaemic but patients should be monitored closely

Target saturation
94–98%

If hypoxaemic (SpO₂ <94%) administer the initial oxygen dose, then adjust oxygen flow to aim for target saturation within the range of **94–98%**, as per the table below.

Condition	Initial dose	Method of administration
• Most poisonings and drug overdoses (refer to **page 144** for **carbon monoxide poisoning** and special cases below for **paraquat poisoning**)	**SpO₂ <85%** 10–15 litres per minute	Reservoir mask (non-rebreathe mask)
• Metabolic and renal disorders • Acute and sub-acute neurological and muscular conditions producing muscle weakness (assess the need for assisted ventilation if **SpO₂ <94%**)	**SpO₂ ≥85–93%** 2–6 litres per minute	Nasal cannulae
• Post convulsion • Gastrointestinal bleeds • Glycaemic emergencies • Heat exhaustion/heat stroke	**SpO₂ ≥85–93%** 5–10 litres per minute	Simple face mask

SPECIAL CASES
• Poisoning with paraquat

NOTE – patients with paraquat poisoning may be harmed by supplemental oxygen so avoid oxygen unless the patient is hypoxaemic. Target saturation 88–92%.

Oxygen   **OXG**

Critical illnesses in adults requiring **HIGH** levels of supplemental oxygen

- Cardiac arrest or resuscitation:
  - basic life support
  - advanced life support
  - foreign body airway obstruction
  - traumatic cardiac arrest
  - maternal resuscitation.
- Major trauma:
  - abdominal trauma
  - burns and scalds
  - electrocution
  - head trauma
  - limb trauma
  - neck and back trauma (spinal)
  - pelvic trauma
  - the immersion incident
  - thoracic trauma
  - trauma in pregnancy.
- Active convulsion
- Anaphylaxis
- Carbon monoxide poisoning
- Hypothermia
- Major pulmonary haemorrhage
- Sepsis e.g. meningococcal septicaemia
- Shock

Oxygen

Serious illnesses in adults requiring MODERATE levels of supplemental oxygen if hypoxaemic

- Acute hypoxaemia
- Deterioration of lung fibrosis or other interstitial lung disease
- Acute asthma
- Acute heart failure
- Pneumonia
- Lung cancer
- Postoperative breathlessness
- Pulmonary embolism
- Pleural effusions
- Pneumothorax
- Severe anaemia
- Sickle cell crisis

Oxygen

OXG

COPD and other conditions in adults requiring **CONTROLLED OR LOW-DOSE** supplemental oxygen

- Chronic Obstructive Pulmonary Disease (COPD)
- Exacerbation of cystic fibrosis
- Chronic neuromuscular disorders
- Chest wall disorders
- Morbid obesity (body mass index >40 kg/m^2)

Oxygen

OXG

Conditions in adults **NOT** requiring supplemental oxygen unless the patient is hypoxaemic

- Myocardial infarction and acute coronary syndromes
- Stroke
- Cardiac rhythm disturbance
- Non-traumatic chest pain/discomfort
- Implantable cardioverter defibrillator firing
- Pregnancy and obstetric emergencies:
    - birth imminent
    - haemorrhage during pregnancy
    - pregnancy induced hypertension
    - vaginal bleeding.
- Abdominal pain
- Headache
- Hyperventilation syndrome or dysfunctional breathing
- Most poisonings and drug overdoses (except carbon monoxide poisoning)
- Metabolic and renal disorders
- Acute and sub-acute neurological and muscular conditions producing muscle weakness
- Post convulsion
- Gastrointestinal bleeds
- Glycaemic emergencies
- Heat exhaustion/heat stroke

Special cases:
- Paraquat poisoning

Oxygen

Is the patient in **CARDIAC** and/or **RESPIRATORY ARREST** or in need of **VENTILATORY SUPPORT?**

YES → Administer the maximum dose of oxygen via a bag-valve-mask until the vital signs are normal, then aim for target saturation within the range of **94–98%**

NO

Do you know or suspect **CARBON MONOXIDE** poisoning?

YES → Administer maximum dose of oxygen via a reservoir mask

NO

Do you know or suspect a critical illness requiring **HIGH** levels of oxygen? **Refer to page 150**

YES → Is SpO$_2$ ≥94% and are the vital signs normal?

NO → Administer 15 l/min of oxygen via a reservoir mask until the vital signs are normal, then aim for target saturation within the range of **94–98%**

YES → Monitor SpO$_2$ and if the saturation falls below **94%** administer oxygen to maintain a saturation within the range of **94–98%**

NO

Do you know or suspect a condition requiring **CONTROLLED OR LOW–DOSE** levels of oxygen? **Refer to page 152**

YES → Is SpO$_2$ ≥88%?

NO → Administer 4 l/min of oxygen via a 28% Venturi mask or patient's own mask to aim for target saturation within the range of **88–92%**

YES → Monitor SpO$_2$ and if the saturation falls below **88%** administer oxygen to maintain a saturation within the range of **88–92%**

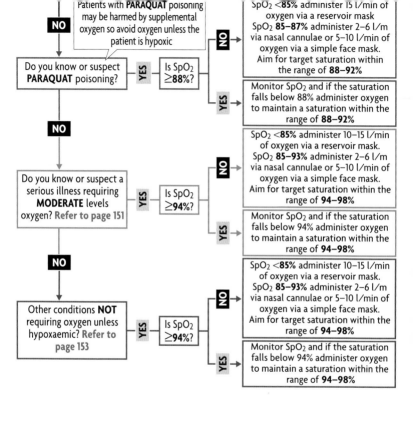

Patients with **PARAQUAT** poisoning may be harmed by supplemental oxygen so avoid oxygen unless the patient is hypoxic

Do you know or suspect **PARAQUAT** poisoning? — **YES** — Is SpO₂ ≥88%?

NO

SpO₂ <85% administer 15 l/min of oxygen via a reservoir mask
SpO₂ 85–87% administer 2–6 l/m via nasal cannulae or 5–10 l/min of oxygen via a simple face mask.
Aim for target saturation within the range of **88–92%**

YES

Monitor SpO₂ and if the saturation falls below 88% administer oxygen to maintain a saturation within the range of **88–92%**

NO

Do you know or suspect a serious illness requiring **MODERATE** levels oxygen? Refer to page 151 — **YES** — Is SpO₂ ≥94%?

NO

SpO₂ <85% administer 10–15 l/min of oxygen via a reservoir mask.
SpO₂ 85–93% administer 2–6 l/m via nasal cannulae or 5–10 l/min of oxygen via a simple face mask.
Aim for target saturation within the range of **94–98%**

YES

Monitor SpO₂ and if the saturation falls below 94% administer oxygen to maintain a saturation within the range of **94–98%**

NO

Other conditions **NOT** requiring oxygen unless hypoxaemic? Refer to page 153 — **YES** — Is SpO₂ ≥94%?

NO

SpO₂ <85% administer 10–15 l/min of oxygen via a reservoir mask.
SpO₂ 85–93% administer 2–6 l/m via nasal cannulae or 5–10 l/min of oxygen via a simple face mask.
Aim for target saturation within the range of **94–98%**

YES

Monitor SpO₂ and if the saturation falls below 94% administer oxygen to maintain a saturation within the range of **94–98%**

Paracetamol

Presentation

Both oral and intravenous preparations are available.

Oral
Paracetamol solutions/suspensions:
- **Infant paracetamol suspension** (120 milligrams in 5 ml), used from 3 months to 5 years.
- **Paracetamol Six Plus Suspension** (250 milligrams in 5 ml), used from 6 years of age upwards.

Paracetamol tablets
- 500 milligram tablets.

Intravenous
- Bottle containing paracetamol 1 gram in 100 ml (10 mg/ml) for intravenous infusion.

Indications

Relief of mild to moderate pain and/or high temperature.

As part of a balanced analgesic regimen for severe pain (IV paracetamol is effective in reducing opioid requirements while improving analgesic efficacy). Only use IV paracetamol for severe pain or if contra-indication to opiates.

Actions

Analgesic (pain relieving) and antipyretic (temperature reducing) drug.

Paracetamol

PAR

Contra-indications

Known paracetamol allergy.

Do **NOT** give further paracetamol if a paracetamol containing product (e.g. Calpol, Co-codamol) has already been given within the last four hours or if the maximum cumulative daily dose has been given already.

Side Effects

Side effects are extremely rare; occasionally intravenous paracetamol may cause systemic hypotension if administered too rapidly.

Additional Information

A febrile child should not be left at home except where:

● a full assessment has been carried out,

and

● the child has no apparent serious underlying illness,

and

● the child has a defined clinical pathway for re-assessment and follow-up, with the full consent of the parent (or carer).

Any IV paracetamol that remains within the giving set can be flushed using 0.9% saline. Take care to ensure that air does not become entrained into the giving set; if there is air in the giving set ensure that it does not run into the patient with further fluids. Ambulance clinicians should stictly adhere to the administration procedure as set out by their Trust to minimise this risk.

Paracetamol

PAR

Dosage and Administration

> **NB** Ensure:
> 1. Paracetamol has not been taken within the previous 4 hours.
> 2. The correct paracetamol containing solution/suspension for the patient's age is being used i.e. 'infant paracetamol suspension' for age groups 0–5 years: 'paracetamol six plus suspension' for ages 6 years and over.

Route: Oral – infant paracetamol suspension.

AGE	INITIAL DOSE	REPEAT DOSE	DOSE INTERVAL	VOLUME	MAXIMUM DOSE
Adult	N/A	N/A	N/A	N/A	N/A
11 years	N/A	N/A	N/A	N/A	N/A
10 years	N/A	N/A	N/A	N/A	N/A
9 years	N/A	N/A	N/A	N/A	N/A
8 years	N/A	N/A	N/A	N/A	N/A
7 years	N/A	N/A	N/A	N/A	N/A
6 years	N/A	N/A	N/A	N/A	N/A
5 years 120 milligrams in 5 ml	240 milligrams	240 milligrams	4–6 hours	10 ml	960 milligrams in 24 hours
4 years 120 milligrams in 5 ml	240 milligrams	240 milligrams	4–6 hours	10 ml	960 milligrams in 24 hours

Paracetamol

Route: Oral – infant paracetamol suspension – *continued.*

AGE	INITIAL DOSE	REPEAT DOSE	DOSE INTERVAL	VOLUME	MAXIMUM DOSE
3 years 120 milligrams in 5 ml	180 milligrams	180 milligrams	4–6 hours	7.5 ml	720 milligrams in 24 hours
2 years 120 milligrams in 5 ml	180 milligrams	180 milligrams	4–6 hours	7.5 ml	720 milligrams in 24 hours
18 months 120 milligrams in 5 ml	120 milligrams	120 milligrams	4–6 hours	5 ml	480 milligrams in 24 hours
12 months 120 milligrams in 5 ml	120 milligrams	120 milligrams	4–6 hours	5 ml	480 milligrams in 24 hours
9 months 120 milligrams in 5 ml	120 milligrams	120 milligrams	4–6 hours	5 ml	480 milligrams in 24 hours
6 months 120 milligrams in 5 ml	120 milligrams	120 milligrams	4–6 hours	5 ml	480 milligrams in 24 hours
3 months 120 milligrams in 5 ml	60 milligrams	60 milligrams	4–6 hours	2.5 ml	240 milligrams in 24 hours
1 month	N/A	N/A	N/A	N/A	N/A
Birth	N/A	N/A	N/A	N/A	N/A

Paracetamol

PAR

> **NB** Ensure:
>
> 1. Paracetamol has not been taken within the previous 4 hours.
> 2. The correct paracetamol containing solution/suspension for the patient's age is being used i.e. 'infant paracetamol suspension' for age groups 0–5 years: 'paracetamol six plus suspension' for ages 6 years and over.

Route: Oral – Paracetamol Six Plus Suspension.

AGE	INITIAL DOSE	REPEAT DOSE	DOSE INTERVAL	VOLUME	MAXIMUM DOSE
12 years – Adult 250 milligrams in 5 ml	1 gram	1 gram	4–6 hours	20 ml	4 grams in 24 hours
11 years 250 milligrams in 5 ml	500 milligrams	500 milligrams	4–6 hours	10 ml	2 grams in 24 hours
10 years 250 milligrams in 5 ml	500 milligrams	500 milligrams	4–6 hours	10 ml	2 grams in 24 hours
9 years 250 milligrams in 5 ml	375 milligrams	375 milligrams	4–6 hours	7.5 ml	1.5 grams in 24 hours
8 years 250 milligrams in 5 ml	375 milligrams	375 milligrams	4–6 hours	7.5 ml	1.5 grams in 24 hours

Paracetamol

PAR

Route: Oral – Paracetamol Six Plus Suspension – *continued.*

AGE	INITIAL DOSE	REPEAT DOSE	DOSE INTERVAL	VOLUME	MAXIMUM DOSE
7 years 250 milligrams in 5 ml	250 milligrams	250 milligrams	4–6 hours	5 ml	1 gram in 24 hours
6 years 250 milligrams in 5 ml	250 milligrams	250 milligrams	4–6 hours	5 ml	1 gram in 24 hours
5 years	N/A	N/A	N/A	N/A	N/A
4 years	N/A	N/A	N/A	N/A	N/A
3 years	N/A	N/A	N/A	N/A	N/A
2 years	N/A	N/A	N/A	N/A	N/A
18 months	N/A	N/A	N/A	N/A	N/A
12 months	N/A	N/A	N/A	N/A	N/A
9 months	N/A	N/A	N/A	N/A	N/A
6 months	N/A	N/A	N/A	N/A	N/A
3 months	N/A	N/A	N/A	N/A	N/A
1 month	N/A	N/A	N/A	N/A	N/A
Birth	N/A	N/A	N/A	N/A	N/A

Paracetamol

PAR

Route: Oral – tablet.

AGE	INITIAL DOSE	REPEAT DOSE	DOSE INTERVAL	VOLUME	MAXIMUM DOSE
12 years – adult 500 milligrams per tablet	1 gram	1 gram	4–6 hours	2 TABLETS	4 grams in 24 hours

NB Ensure:
Paracetamol has not been taken within the previous 4 hours.

Route: Intravenous infusion; typically given over 5–10 minutes.

AGE	INITIAL DOSE	REPEAT DOSE	DOSE INTERVAL	VOLUME	MAXIMUM DOSE
12 years – adult 10 milligrams in 1 ml	1 gram	1 gram	4–6 hours	100 ml	4 grams in 24 hours
11 years 10 milligrams in 1 ml	500 milligrams	500 milligrams	4–6 hours	50 ml	2 grams in 24 hours
10 years 10 milligrams in 1 ml	500 milligrams	500 milligrams	4–6 hours	50 ml	2 grams in 24 hours

Paracetamol

Route: Intravenous infusion; typically given over 5–10 minutes – *continued*.

AGE	INITIAL DOSE	REPEAT DOSE	DOSE INTERVAL	VOLUME	MAXIMUM DOSE
9 years 10 milligrams in 1 ml	500 milligrams	500 milligrams	4–6 hours	50 ml	2 grams in 24 hours
8 years 10 milligrams in 1 ml	300 milligrams	300 milligrams	4–6 hours	30 ml	1.2 grams in 24 hours
7 years 10 milligrams in 1 ml	300 milligrams	300 milligrams	4–6 hours	30 ml	1.2 grams in 24 hours
6 years 10 milligrams in 1 ml	300 milligrams	300 milligrams	4–6 hours	30 ml	1.2 grams in 24 hours
5 years 10 milligrams in 1 ml	250 milligrams	250 milligrams	4–6 hours	25 ml	1 gram in 24 hours
4 years 10 milligrams in 1 ml	250 milligrams	250 milligrams	4–6 hours	25 ml	1 gram in 24 hours
3 years 10 milligrams in 1 ml	250 milligrams	250 milligrams	4–6 hours	25 ml	1 gram in 24 hours
2 years 10 milligrams in 1 ml	125 milligrams	125 milligrams	4–6 hours	12.5 ml	500 in milligrams in 24 hours

Paracetamol

PAR

Route: Intravenous infusion; typically given over 5–10 minutes – *continued*.

AGE	INITIAL DOSE	REPEAT DOSE	DOSE INTERVAL	VOLUME	MAXIMUM DOSE
18 months 10 milligrams in 1 ml	125 milligrams	125 milligrams	4–6 hours	12.5 ml	500 milligrams in 24 hours
12 months 10 milligrams in 1 ml	125 milligrams	125 milligrams	4–6 hours	12.5 ml	500 milligrams in 24 hours
9 months 10 milligrams in 1 ml	50 milligrams	50 milligrams	4–6 hours	5 ml	200 milligrams in 24 hours
6 months 10 milligrams in 1 ml	50 milligrams	50 milligrams	4–6 hours	5 ml	200 milligrams in 24 hours
3 months	N/A	N/A	N/A	N/A	N/A
1 month	N/A	N/A	N/A	N/A	N/A
Birth	N/A	N/A	N/A	N/A	N/A

Reteplase

Presentation

Vials of **reteplase** 10 units for reconstitution with 10 ml water for injection.

NOTE: Whilst the strength of thrombolytics is traditionally expressed in 'units', these units are unique to each particular drug and are **NOT** interchangeable.

Indications

Acute ST segment elevation MI (STEMI) 12 hours of symptom onset where primary percutaneous coronary intervention (PPCI) is **NOT** readily available.

Ensure patient fulfils the criteria for drug administration following the local protocols. Variation of these criteria is justifiable at local level with agreement of appropriate key stakeholders (e.g. cardiac network, or in the context of an approved clinical trial).

Contra-indications

Refer to local Trust checklist for thrombolytics.

Actions

Activates the fibrinolytic system, inducing the breaking up of intravascular thrombi and emboli.

Side Effects

Bleeding:

- major – seek medical advice and transport to hospital rapidly
- minor e.g. at injection sites – use local pressure.

Reteplase

Arhythmias – these are usually benign in the form of transient idioventricular rhythms and usually require no special treatment. Treat ventricular fibrillation (VF) as a complication of myocardial infarction (MI) with standard protocols; bradycardia with atropine as required.

Anaphylaxis – extremely rare (0.1%) with third generation bolus agents.

Hypotension – often responds to laying the patient flat.

Additional Information

PPCI is now the dominant reperfusion treatment and should be used where available; patients with STEMI will be taken direct to a specialist cardiac centre instead of receiving thrombolysis (**refer to acute coronary syndrome guideline**). Local protocol should be followed.

'Time is muscle!' Do not delay transportation to hospital if difficulties arise whilst setting up the equipment or establishing IV access. Qualified single responders should administer a thrombolytic if indicated while awaiting arrival of an ambulance.

In All Cases

Ensure a defibrillator is immediately available at all times.

Monitor conscious level, pulse, blood pressure and cardiac rhythm during and following injections. Manage complications (associated with the acute MI) as they occur using standard protocols. The main early adverse event associated with thrombolysis is bleeding, which should be managed according to standard protocols.

AT HOSPITAL – emphasise the need to commence a heparin infusion in accordance with local protocols – to reduce the risk of re-infarction.

Reteplase

Dosage and Administration

RETEPLASE

1. Administer a bolus of intravenous injection un-fractionated heparin before the first dose of reteplase (**refer to heparin guideline**). Flush the cannula well with saline **OR** use a separate cannula to administer reteplase as the two agents are physically incompatible.

2. Note the time the first dose is administered.

3. Administer the second dose 30 minutes after the first.

4. **AT HOSPITAL** – It is essential that the care of the patient is handed over as soon as possible to a member of hospital staff qualified to administer the second bolus (if not already given) and commence a heparin infusion.

Route: Intravenous bolus injections separated by 30 minutes.

AGE	INITIAL DOSE	REPEAT DOSE	DOSE INTERVAL	VOLUME	MAXIMUM DOSE
≥18 10 units in 10 ml	First dose 10 units	NONE	N/A	10 ml	10 units
	Second dose 10 units	NONE	N/A	10 ml	10 units

Salbutamol

SLB

Presentation

Nebules containing salbutamol 2.5 milligrams/2.5 ml or
5 milligrams/2.5 ml.

Indications

Acute asthma attack where normal inhaler therapy has failed to relieve
symptoms.

Expiratory wheezing associated with allergy, anaphylaxis, smoke
inhalation or other lower airway cause.

Exacerbation of chronic obstructive pulmonary disease (COPD).

Shortness of breath in patients with severe breathing difficulty due to
left ventricular failure (secondary treatment).

Actions

Salbutamol is a selective beta2 adrenoreceptor stimulant drug. This has a
relaxant effect on the smooth muscle in the medium and smaller
airways, which are in spasm in acute asthma attacks. If given by nebuliser,
especially if oxygen powered, its smooth-muscle relaxing action,
combined with the airway moistening effect of nebulisation, can relieve
the attack rapidly.

Contra-indications

None in the emergency situation.

Salbutamol

Cautions

Salbutamol should be used with care in patients with:

- Hypertension.
- Angina.
- Overactive thyroid.
- Late pregnancy (can relax uterus).
- Severe hypertension may occur in patients on beta-blockers and half doses should be used unless there is profound hypotension.

If COPD is a possibility limit nebulisation to six minutes.

Side Effects

Tremor (shaking).

Tachycardia.

Palpitations.

Headache.

Feeling of tension.

Peripheral vasodilatation.

Muscle cramps.

Rash.

Additional Information

In acute severe or life-threatening asthma ipratropium should be given after the first dose of salbutamol. In acute asthma or COPD unresponsive to salbutamol alone, a single dose of ipratropium may be given after salbutamol.

Salbutamol

SLB

Salbutamol often provides initial relief. In more severe attacks however, the use of steroids by injection or orally and further nebuliser therapy will be required. Do not be lulled into a false sense of security by an initial improvement after salbutamol nebulisation.

Dosage and Administration

- **In life-threatening or acute severe asthma:** undertake a **TIME CRITICAL** transfer to the **NEAREST SUITABLE RECEIVING HOSPITAL** and provide nebulisation en route.
- If COPD is a possibility limit nebulisation to six minutes.
- The pulse rate in children may exceed 140 after significant doses of salbutamol; this is not usually of any clinical significance and should not usually preclude further use of the drug.
- Repeat doses should be discontinued if the side effects are becoming significant (e.g. tremors, tachycardia >140 beats per minute in adults) – this is a clinical decision by the ambulance clinician.

Route: Nebulised with 6–8 litres per minute of oxygen.

AGE	INITIAL DOSE	REPEAT DOSE	DOSE INTERVAL	VOLUME	MAXIMUM DOSE
Adult 2.5 milligrams in 2.5 ml	5 milligrams	5 milligrams	5 minutes	5 ml	No limit

Salbutamol

Route: Nebulised with 6–8 litres per minute of oxygen.

AGE	INITIAL DOSE	REPEAT DOSE	DOSE INTERVAL	VOLUME	MAXIMUM DOSE
Adult 5 milligrams in 2.5 ml	5 milligrams	5 milligrams	5 minutes	2.5 ml	No limit

0.9% Sodium Chloride

Presentation

100 ml, 250 ml, 500 ml and 1,000 ml packs of sodium chloride intravenous infusion 0.9%.

5 ml and 10 ml ampoules for use as flushes.

5 ml and 10 ml pre-loaded syringes for use as flushes.

Indications

Adult Fluid Therapy

- Medical conditions without haemorrhage.
- Medical conditions with haemorrhage.
- Trauma related haemorrhage.
- Burns.
- Limb crush injury.

Child Fluid Therapy

- Medical conditions.
- Trauma related haemorrhage.
- Burns.

Flush

- As a flush to confirm patency of an intravenous or intra-osseous cannula.
- As a flush following drug administration.

0.9% Sodium Chloride

Actions

Increases vascular fluid volume which consequently raises cardiac output and improves perfusion.

Contra-indications

None.

Side Effects

Over-infusion may precipitate pulmonary oedema and cause breathlessness.

Additional Information

Fluid replacement in cases of dehydration should occur over hours; rapid fluid replacement is seldom indicated; **refer to intravascular fluid therapy guidelines**.

Dosage and Administration

Route: Intravenous or Intra-osseous for **ALL** conditions.

FLUSH

AGE	INITIAL DOSE	REPEAT DOSE	DOSE INTERVAL	VOLUME	MAXIMUM DOSE
Adult 0.9%	2 ml – 5 ml	2 ml – 5 ml	PRN	2 – 5 ml	N/A
Adult 0.9%	10 ml – 20 ml (if infusing glucose)	10 ml – 20 ml if infusing glucose	PRN	10 – 20 ml	N/A

0.9% Sodium Chloride   **SCP**

ADULT MEDICAL EMERGENCIES

General medical conditions without haemorrhage: Anaphylaxis, hyperglycaemic ketoacidosis, dehydration*

AGE	INITIAL DOSE	REPEAT DOSE	DOSE INTERVAL	VOLUME	MAXIMUM DOSE
Adult 0.9%	250 ml	250 ml	PRN	250 ml	2 litres

Sepsis: Clinical signs of infection **AND** systolic BP<90 mmHg **AND** tachypnoea

AGE	INITIAL DOSE	REPEAT DOSE	DOSE INTERVAL	VOLUME	MAXIMUM DOSE
Adult 0.9%	1 litre	1 litre	30 minutes	1 litre	2 litres

Medical conditions with haemorrhage: Systolic BP<90 mmHg and signs of poor perfusion

AGE	INITIAL DOSE	REPEAT DOSE	DOSE INTERVAL	VOLUME	MAXIMUM DOSE
Adult 0.9%	250 ml	250 ml	PRN	250 ml	2 litres

*In cases of dehydration fluid replacement should usually occur over hours.

0.9% Sodium Chloride SCP

ADULT TRAUMA EMERGENCIES

Blunt trauma, head trauma or penetrating limb trauma: Systolic BP<90 mmHg and signs of poor perfusion

AGE	INITIAL DOSE	REPEAT DOSE	DOSE INTERVAL	VOLUME	MAXIMUM DOSE
Adult 0.9%	250 ml	250 ml	PRN	250 ml	2 litres

Penetrating torso trauma: Systolic BP<60 mmHg and signs of poor perfusion

AGE	INITIAL DOSE	REPEAT DOSE	DOSE INTERVAL	VOLUME	MAXIMUM DOSE
Adult 0.9%	250 ml	250 ml	PRN	250 ml	2 litres

Burns:

- Total body surface area (TBSA): between 15% and 25% and time to hospital is greater than 30 minutes.
- TBSA: more than 25%.

AGE	INITIAL DOSE	REPEAT DOSE	DOSE INTERVAL	VOLUME	MAXIMUM DOSE
Adult 0.9%	1 litre	NONE	N/A	1 litre	1 litre

0.9% Sodium Chloride   SCP

Limb crush injury

AGE	INITIAL DOSE	REPEAT DOSE	DOSE INTERVAL	VOLUME	MAXIMUM DOSE
Adult 0.9%	2 litres	NONE	N/A	2 litres	2 litres

NB Manage crush injury of the torso as per blunt trauma.

0.9% Sodium Chloride SCP

MEDICAL EMERGENCIES IN CHILDREN (20 ml/kg)
NB Exceptions: cardiac failure, renal failure, diabetic ketoacidosis (see following).

AGE	INITIAL DOSE	REPEAT DOSE	DOSE INTERVAL	VOLUME	MAXIMUM DOSE
11 years 0.9%	500 ml	500 ml	PRN	500 ml	1000 ml
10 years 0.9%	500 ml	500 ml	PRN	500 ml	1000 ml
9 years 0.9%	500 ml	500 ml	PRN	500 ml	1000 ml
8 years 0.9%	500 ml	500 ml	PRN	500 ml	1000 ml
7 years 0.9%	460 ml	460 ml	PRN	460 ml	920 ml
6 years 0.9%	420 ml	420 ml	PRN	420 ml	840 ml
5 years 0.9%	380 ml	380 ml	PRN	380 ml	760 ml
4 years 0.9%	320 ml	320 ml	PRN	320 ml	640 ml
3 years 0.9%	280 ml	280 ml	PRN	280 ml	560 ml
2 years 0.9%	240 ml	240 ml	PRN	240 ml	480 ml
18 months 0.9%	220 ml	220 ml	PRN	220 ml	440 ml

0.9% Sodium Chloride SCP

MEDICAL EMERGENCIES IN CHILDREN (20 ml/kg) – *continued*.
NB Exceptions: cardiac failure, renal failure, diabetic ketoacidosis (see following).

AGE	INITIAL DOSE	REPEAT DOSE	DOSE INTERVAL	VOLUME	MAXIMUM DOSE
12 months 0.9%	200 ml	200 ml	PRN	200 ml	400 ml
9 months 0.9%	180 ml	180 ml	PRN	180 ml	360 ml
6 months 0.9%	160 ml	160 ml	PRN	160 ml	320 ml
3 months 0.9%	120 ml	120 ml	PRN	120 ml	240 ml
1 month 0.9%	90 ml	90 ml	PRN	90 ml	180 ml
Birth 0.9%	70 ml	70 ml	PRN	70 ml	140 ml

0.9% Sodium Chloride

MEDICAL EMERGENCIES IN CHILDREN
Heart failure or renal failure (10 ml/kg)

AGE	INITIAL DOSE	REPEAT DOSE	DOSE INTERVAL	VOLUME	MAXIMUM DOSE
11 years 0.9%	350 ml	350 ml	PRN	350 ml	700 ml
10 years 0.9%	320 ml	320 ml	PRN	320 ml	640 ml
9 years 0.9%	290 ml	290 ml	PRN	290 ml	580 ml
8 years 0.9%	250 ml	250 ml	PRN	250 ml	500 ml
7 years 0.9%	230 ml	230 ml	PRN	230 ml	460 ml
6 years 0.9%	210 ml	210 ml	PRN	210 ml	420 ml
5 years 0.9%	190 ml	190 ml	PRN	190 ml	380 ml
4 years 0.9%	160 ml	160 ml	PRN	160 ml	320 ml
3 years 0.9%	140 ml	140 ml	PRN	140 ml	280 ml
2 years 0.9%	120 ml	120 ml	PRN	120 ml	240 ml
18 months 0.9%	110 ml	110 ml	PRN	110 ml	220 ml

RESUS GENERAL MEDICAL TRAUMA SP SITU PAED DRUGS PAGE AGE 179

0.9% Sodium Chloride

SCP

MEDICAL EMERGENCIES IN CHILDREN – *continued.*
Heart failure or renal failure (10 ml/kg)

AGE	INITIAL DOSE	REPEAT DOSE	DOSE INTERVAL	VOLUME	MAXIMUM DOSE
12 months 0.9%	100 ml	100 ml	PRN	100 ml	200 ml
9 months 0.9%	90 ml	90 ml	PRN	90 ml	180 ml
6 months 0.9%	80 ml	80 ml	PRN	80 ml	160 ml
3 months 0.9%	60 ml	60 ml	PRN	60 ml	120 ml
1 month 0.9%	45 ml	45 ml	PRN	45 ml	90 ml
Birth 0.9%	35 ml	35 ml	PRN	35 ml	70 ml

0.9% Sodium Chloride

SCP

MEDICAL EMERGENCIES IN CHILDREN
Diabetic ketoacidosis (10 ml/kg) administer **ONCE** only over 15 minutes.

AGE	INITIAL DOSE	REPEAT DOSE	DOSE INTERVAL	VOLUME	MAXIMUM DOSE
11 years 0.9%	350 ml	NONE	N/A	350 ml	350 ml
10 years 0.9%	320 ml	NONE	N/A	320 ml	320 ml
9 years 0.9%	290 ml	NONE	N/A	290 ml	290 ml
8 years 0.9%	250 ml	NONE	N/A	250 ml	250 ml
7 years 0.9%	230 ml	NONE	N/A	230 ml	230 ml
6 years 0.9%	210 ml	NONE	N/A	210 ml	210 ml
5 years 0.9%	190 ml	NONE	N/A	190 ml	190 ml
4 years 0.9%	160 ml	NONE	N/A	160 ml	160 ml
3 years 0.9%	140 ml	NONE	N/A	140 ml	140 ml
2 years 0.9%	120 ml	NONE	N/A	120 ml	120 ml
18 months 0.9%	110 ml	NONE	N/A	110 ml	110 ml

0.9% Sodium Chloride

MEDICAL EMERGENCIES IN CHILDREN – *continued.*
Diabetic ketoacidosis (10 ml/kg) administer **ONCE** only over 15 minutes.

AGE	INITIAL DOSE	REPEAT DOSE	DOSE INTERVAL	VOLUME	MAXIMUM DOSE
12 months 0.9%	100 ml	NONE	N/A	100 ml	100 ml
9 months 0.9%	90 ml	NONE	N/A	90 ml	90 ml
6 months 0.9%	80 ml	NONE	N/A	80 ml	80 ml
3 months 0.9%	60 ml	NONE	N/A	60 ml	60 ml
1 month 0.9%	45 ml	NONE	N/A	45 ml	45 ml
Birth 0.9%	35 ml	NONE	N/A	35 ml	35 ml

0.9% Sodium Chloride

SCP

TRAUMA EMERGENCIES IN CHILDREN (5 ml/kg)

NB Exceptions: burns.

AGE	INITIAL DOSE	REPEAT DOSE	DOSE INTERVAL	VOLUME	MAXIMUM DOSE
11 years 0.9%	175 ml	175 ml	PRN	175 ml	1000 ml
10 years 0.9%	160 ml	160 ml	PRN	160 ml	1000 ml
9 years 0.9%	145 ml	145 ml	PRN	145 ml	1000 ml
8 years 0.9%	130 ml	130 ml	PRN	130 ml	1000 ml
7 years 0.9%	115 ml	115 ml	PRN	115 ml	920 ml
6 years 0.9%	105 ml	105 ml	PRN	105 ml	840 ml
5 years 0.9%	95 ml	95 ml	PRN	95 ml	760 ml
4 years 0.9%	80 ml	80 ml	PRN	80 ml	640 ml
3 years 0.9%	70 ml	70 ml	PRN	70 ml	560 ml
2 years 0.9%	60 ml	60 ml	PRN	60 ml	480 ml
18 months 0.9%	55 ml	55 ml	PRN	55 ml	440 ml

0.9% Sodium Chloride

SCP

TRAUMA EMERGENCIES IN CHILDREN (5 ml/kg) – *continued.*

NB Exceptions: burns.

AGE	INITIAL DOSE	REPEAT DOSE	DOSE INTERVAL	VOLUME	MAXIMUM DOSE
12 months 0.9%	50 ml	50 ml	PRN	50 ml	400 ml
9 months 0.9%	45 ml	45 ml	PRN	45 ml	360 ml
6 months 0.9%	40 ml	40 ml	PRN	40 ml	320 ml
3 months 0.9%	30 ml	30 ml	PRN	30 ml	240 ml
1 month 0.9%	20 ml	20 ml	PRN	20 ml	180 ml
Birth 0.9%	20 ml	20 ml	PRN	20 ml	140 ml

0.9% Sodium Chloride

SCP

Burns (10 ml/kg, given over 1 hour):

- TBSA: between 10% and 20% and time to hospital is greater than 30 minutes.
- TBSA: more than 20%.

AGE	INITIAL DOSE	REPEAT DOSE	DOSE INTERVAL	VOLUME	MAXIMUM DOSE
11 years 0.9%	350 ml	NONE	N/A	350 ml	350 ml
10 years 0.9%	320 ml	NONE	N/A	320 ml	320 ml
9 years 0.9%	290 ml	NONE	N/A	290 ml	290 ml
8 years 0.9%	250 ml	NONE	N/A	250 ml	250 ml
7 years 0.9%	230 ml	NONE	N/A	230 ml	230 ml
6 years 0.9%	210 ml	NONE	N/A	210 ml	210 ml
5 years 0.9%	190 ml	NONE	N/A	190 ml	190 ml
4 years 0.9%	160 ml	NONE	N/A	160 ml	160 ml
3 years 0.9%	140 ml	NONE	N/A	140 ml	140 ml
2 years 0.9%	120 ml	NONE	N/A	120 ml	120 ml

0.9% Sodium Chloride

SCP

Burns (10 ml/kg, given over 1 hour) – *continued.*

- TBSA: between 10% and 20% and time to hospital is greater than 30 minutes.
- TBSA: more than 20%.

AGE	INITIAL DOSE	REPEAT DOSE	DOSE INTERVAL	VOLUME	MAXIMUM DOSE
18 months 0.9%	110 ml	NONE	N/A	110 ml	110 ml
12 months 0.9%	100 ml	NONE	N/A	100 ml	100 ml
9 months 0.9%	90 ml	NONE	N/A	90 ml	90 ml
6 months 0.9%	80 ml	NONE	N/A	80 ml	80 ml
3 months 0.9%	60 ml	NONE	N/A	60 ml	60 ml
1 month 0.9%	45 ml	NONE	N/A	45 ml	45 ml
Birth 0.9%	35 ml	NONE	N/A	35 ml	35 ml

Sodium Lactate Compound (Hartmann's/Ringer's Lactate)

SLC

Presentation

250 ml, 500 ml and 1,000 ml packs of compound sodium lactate intravenous infusion (also called Hartmann's solution for injection or Ringer's-Lactate solution for injection).

Indications

Blood and fluid loss, to correct hypovolaemia and improve tissue perfusion if sodium chloride 0.9% is **NOT** available.

Dehydration.

Actions

Increases vascular fluid volume which consequently raises cardiac output and improves perfusion.

Contra-indications

Diabetic hyperglycaemic ketoacidotic coma, and pre-coma.
NB Administer 0.9% sodium chloride intravenous infusion.

Neonates.

Cautions

Sodium lactate should not be used in limb crush injury when 0.9% sodium chloride is available.

Renal failure.

Liver failure.

Sodium Lactate Compound (Hartmann's/Ringer's Lactate)

SLC

Side Effects

Infusion of an excessive volume may overload the circulation and precipitate heart failure (increased breathlessness, wheezing and distended neck veins). Volume overload is unlikely if the patient is correctly assessed initially and it is very unlikely indeed if patient response is assessed after initial 250 ml infusion and then after each 250 ml of infusion. If there is evidence of this complication, the patient should be transported rapidly to nearest suitable receiving hospital whilst administering high-flow oxygen.

Do not administer further fluid.

Additional Information

Compound sodium lactate intravenous infusion contains mainly sodium, but also small amounts of potassium and lactate. It is useful for initial fluid replacement in cases of blood loss.

The volume of compound sodium lactate intravenous infusion needed is 3 times as great as the volume of blood loss. Sodium lactate has **NO** oxygen carrying capacity.

Sodium Lactate Compound (Hartmann's/Ringer's Lactate) SLC

Dosage and Administration if sodium chloride 0.9% is NOT available.

Route: Intravenous or intra-osseous for **ALL** conditions.

ADULT MEDICAL EMERGENCIES

General medical conditions without haemorrhage: anaphylaxis, dehydration*.

NB Exception sodium lactate compound is contra-indicated in diabetic ketoacidosis – **refer to sodium chloride 0.9% guideline**.

AGE	INITIAL DOSE	REPEAT DOSE	DOSE INTERVAL	VOLUME	MAXIMUM DOSE
Adult Compound	250 ml	250 ml	PRN	250 ml	2 litres

Sepsis: Clinical signs of infection **AND** systolic BP<90 mmHg **AND** tachypnoea

AGE	INITIAL DOSE	REPEAT DOSE	DOSE INTERVAL	VOLUME	MAXIMUM DOSE
Adult Compound	1 litre	1 litre	30 minutes	1 litre	2 litres

*In cases of dehydration fluid replacement should usually occur over hours.

Sodium Lactate Compound (Hartmann's/Ringer's Lactate)   SLC

ADULT TRAUMA EMERGENCIES

Medical conditions with haemorrhage: Systolic BP<90 mmHg and signs of poor perfusion.

AGE	INITIAL DOSE	REPEAT DOSE	DOSE INTERVAL	VOLUME	MAXIMUM DOSE
Adult Compound	250 ml	250 ml	PRN	250 ml	2 litres

Blunt trauma, head trauma or penetrating limb trauma: Systolic BP<90 mmHg and signs of poor perfusion.

AGE	INITIAL DOSE	REPEAT DOSE	DOSE INTERVAL	VOLUME	MAXIMUM DOSE
Adult Compound	250 ml	250 ml	PRN	250 ml	2 litres

Penetrating torso trauma: Systolic BP<60 mmHg and signs of poor perfusion.

AGE	INITIAL DOSE	REPEAT DOSE	DOSE INTERVAL	VOLUME	MAXIMUM DOSE
Adult Compound	250 ml	250 ml	PRN	250 ml	2 litres

Sodium Lactate Compound   SLC
(Hartmann's/Ringer's Lactate)

Burns:

- TBSA: between 15% and 25% and time to hospital is greater than 30 minutes.
- TBSA: more than 25%.

AGE	INITIAL DOSE	REPEAT DOSE	DOSE INTERVAL	VOLUME	MAXIMUM DOSE
Adult Compound	1 litre	N/A	N/A	1 litre	1 litre

Limb crush injury

AGE	INITIAL DOSE	REPEAT DOSE	DOSE INTERVAL	VOLUME	MAXIMUM DOSE
Adult Compound	2 litres	N/A	N/A	2 litres	2 litres

NB Sodium chloride 0.9% is the fluid of choice in crush injury.
NB Manage crush injury of the torso as per blunt trauma.

Sodium Lactate Compound (Hartmann's/Ringer's Lactate)   SLC

MEDICAL EMERGENCIES IN CHILDREN (20 ml/kg) – **NB** Exceptions heart failure, renal failure, liver failure, diabetic ketoacidosis (sodium lactate compound is contra-indicated in diabetic ketoacidosis – **refer to sodium chloride 0.9% guideline**).

AGE	INITIAL DOSE	REPEAT DOSE	DOSE INTERVAL	VOLUME	MAXIMUM DOSE
11 years Compound	500 ml	500 ml	PRN	500 ml	1 litre
10 years Compound	500 ml	500 ml	PRN	500 ml	1 litre
9 years Compound	500 ml	500 ml	PRN	500 ml	1 litre
8 years Compound	500 ml	500 ml	PRN	500 ml	1000 ml
7 years Compound	460 ml	460 ml	PRN	460 ml	920 ml
6 years Compound	420 ml	420 ml	PRN	420 ml	840 ml
5 years Compound	380 ml	380 ml	PRN	380 ml	760 ml
4 years Compound	320 ml	320 ml	PRN	320 ml	640 ml
3 years Compound	280 ml	280 ml	PRN	280 ml	560 ml

Sodium Lactate Compound (Hartmann's/Ringer's Lactate) SLC

MEDICAL EMERGENCIES IN CHILDREN (20 ml/kg) – NB Exceptions heart failure, renal failure, liver failure, diabetic ketoacidosis (sodium lactate compound is contra-indicated in diabetic ketoacidosis (**refer to sodium chloride 0.9% guideline**) – *continued*.

AGE	INITIAL DOSE	REPEAT DOSE	DOSE INTERVAL	VOLUME	MAXIMUM DOSE
2 years Compound	240 ml	240 ml	PRN	240 ml	480 ml
18 months Compound	220 ml	220 ml	PRN	220 ml	440 ml
12 months Compound	200 ml	200 ml	PRN	200 ml	400 ml
9 months Compound	180 ml	180 ml	PRN	180 ml	360 ml
6 months Compound	160 ml	160 ml	PRN	160 ml	320 ml
3 months Compound	120 ml	120 ml	PRN	120 ml	240 ml
1 month Compound	90 ml	90 ml	PRN	90 ml	180 ml
Birth N/A	N/A	N/A	N/A	N/A	N/A

Sodium Lactate Compound (Hartmann's/Ringer's Lactate)   SLC

MEDICAL EMERGENCIES IN CHILDREN

Heart failure or renal failure (10 ml/kg)

AGE	INITIAL DOSE	REPEAT DOSE	DOSE INTERVAL	VOLUME	MAXIMUM DOSE
11 years Compound	350 ml	350 ml	PRN	350 ml	700 ml
10 years Compound	320 ml	320 ml	PRN	320 ml	640 ml
9 years Compound	290 ml	290 ml	PRN	290 ml	580 ml
8 years Compound	250 ml	250 ml	PRN	250 ml	500 ml
7 years Compound	230 ml	230 ml	PRN	230 ml	460 ml
6 years Compound	210 ml	210 ml	PRN	210 ml	420 ml
5 years Compound	190 ml	190 ml	PRN	190 ml	380 ml
4 years Compound	160 ml	160 ml	PRN	160 ml	320 ml
3 years Compound	140 ml	140 ml	PRN	140 ml	280 ml
2 years Compound	120 ml	120 ml	PRN	120 ml	240 ml

Sodium Lactate Compound (Hartmann's/Ringer's Lactate)   SLC

MEDICAL EMERGENCIES IN CHILDREN

Heart failure or renal failure (10 ml/kg) – *continued.*

AGE	INITIAL DOSE	REPEAT DOSE	DOSE INTERVAL	VOLUME	MAXIMUM DOSE
18 months Compound	110 ml	110 ml	PRN	110 ml	220 ml
12 months Compound	100 ml	100 ml	PRN	100 ml	200 ml
9 months Compound	90 ml	90 ml	PRN	90 ml	180 ml
6 months Compound	80 ml	80 ml	PRN	80 ml	160 ml
3 months Compound	60 ml	60 ml	PRN	60 ml	120 ml
1 month Compound	45 ml	45 ml	PRN	45 ml	90 ml
Birth Compound	N/A	N/A	N/A	N/A	N/A

Sodium Lactate Compound (Hartmann's/Ringer's Lactate)   SLC

TRAUMA EMERGENCIES IN CHILDREN (5 ml/kg)

NB Exceptions: burns.

AGE	INITIAL DOSE	REPEAT DOSE	DOSE INTERVAL	VOLUME	MAXIMUM DOSE
11 years Compound	175 ml	175 ml	PRN	175 ml	1 litre
10 years Compound	160 ml	160 ml	PRN	160 ml	1 litre
9 years Compound	145 ml	145 ml	PRN	145 ml	1 litre
8 years Compound	130 ml	130 ml	PRN	130 ml	1 litre
7 years Compound	115 ml	115 ml	PRN	115 ml	920 ml
6 years Compound	105 ml	105 ml	PRN	105 ml	840 ml
5 years Compound	95 ml	95 ml	PRN	95 ml	760 ml
4 years Compound	80 ml	80 ml	PRN	80 ml	640 ml
3 years Compound	70 ml	70 ml	PRN	70 ml	560 ml
2 years Compound	60 ml	60 ml	PRN	60 ml	480 m

Sodium Lactate Compound SLC
(Hartmann's/Ringer's Lactate)

TRAUMA EMERGENCIES IN CHILDREN (5 ml/kg)

NB Exceptions: burns – *continued*.

AGE	INITIAL DOSE	REPEAT DOSE	DOSE INTERVAL	VOLUME	MAXIMUM DOSE
18 months Compound	55 ml	55 ml	PRN	55 ml	440 ml
12 months Compound	50 ml	50 ml	PRN	50 ml	400 ml
9 months Compound	45 ml	45 ml	PRN	45 ml	360 ml
6 months Compound	40 ml	40 ml	PRN	40 ml	320 ml
3 months Compound	30 ml	30 ml	PRN	30 ml	240 ml
1 month Compound	20 ml	20 ml	PRN	20 ml	180 ml
Birth N/A	N/A	N/A	N/A	N/A	N/A

Sodium Lactate Compound (Hartmann's/Ringer's Lactate)   SLC

Burns (10 ml/kg, given over 1 hour):

- TBSA: between 10% and 20% and time to hospital is greater than 30 minutes.
- TBSA: more than 20%.

AGE	INITIAL DOSE	REPEAT DOSE	DOSE INTERVAL	VOLUME	MAXIMUM DOSE
11 years Compound	350 ml	NONE	N/A	350 ml	350 ml
10 years Compound	320 ml	NONE	N/A	320 ml	320 ml
9 years Compound	290 ml	NONE	N/A	290 ml	290 ml
8 years Compound	250 ml	NONE	N/A	250 ml	250 ml
7 years Compound	230 ml	NONE	N/A	230 ml	230 ml
6 years Compound	210 ml	NONE	N/A	210 ml	210 ml
5 years Compound	190 ml	NONE	N/A	190 ml	190 ml
4 years Compound	160 ml	NONE	N/A	160 ml	160 ml
3 years Compound	140 ml	NONE	N/A	140 ml	140 ml

Sodium Lactate Compound (Hartmann's/Ringer's Lactate)   SLC

Burns (10 ml/kg, given over 1 hour):

- TBSA: between 10% and 20% and time to hospital is greater than 30 minutes.
- TBSA: more than 20% – *continued*.

AGE	INITIAL DOSE	REPEAT DOSE	DOSE INTERVAL	VOLUME	MAXIMUM DOSE
2 years Compound	120 ml	NONE	N/A	120 ml	120 ml
18 months Compound	110 ml	NONE	N/A	110 ml	110 ml
12 months Compound	100 ml	NONE	N/A	100 ml	100 ml
9 months Compound	90 ml	NONE	N/A	90 ml	90 ml
6 months Compound	80 ml	NONE	N/A	80 ml	80 ml
3 months Compound	60 ml	NONE	N/A	60 ml	60 ml
1 month Compound	45 ml	NONE	N/A	45 ml	45 ml
Birth N/A	N/A	N/A	N/A	N/A	N/A

Syntometrine

Presentation

An ampoule containing ergometrine 500 micrograms and oxytocin 5 units in 1 ml.

Indications

Postpartum haemorrhage within 24 hours of delivery of the infant where bleeding from the uterus is uncontrollable by uterine massage.

Miscarriage with life-threatening bleeding and a confirmed diagnosis e.g. where a patient has gone home with medical management and starts to bleed.

Actions

Stimulates contraction of the uterus.

Onset of action 7–10 minutes.

Contra-indications

- Known hypersensitivity to syntometrine.
- Active labour.
- Severe cardiac, liver or kidney disease.
- Hypertension and severe pre-eclampsia.
- Possible multiple pregnancy/known or suspected fetus in utero.

Syntometrine

SYN

Side Effects

- Nausea and vomiting.
- Abdominal pain.
- Headache.
- Hypertension and bradycardia.
- Chest pain and, rarely, anaphylactic reactions.

Additional Information

Syntometrine and misoprostol reduce bleeding from a pregnant uterus through different pathways; therefore if one drug has not been effective after 15 mins, the other may be administered in addition.

Dosage and Administration

Route: Intramuscular.

AGE	INITIAL DOSE	REPEAT DOSE	DOSE INTERVAL	VOLUME	MAXIMUM DOSE
Adult 500 micrograms of ergometrine and 5 units of oxytocin in 1 ml.	500 micrograms of ergometrine and 5 units of oxytocin.	None	N/A	1 ml	500 micrograms of ergometrine and 5 units of oxytocin.

Tenecteplase

TNK

Presentation

Vials of **tenecteplase** 10,000 units for reconstitution with 10 ml water for injection, or 8,000 units for reconstitution with 8 ml water for injection.

NOTE: Whilst the strength of thrombolytics is traditionally expressed in 'units' these units are unique to each particular drug and are **NOT** interchangeable.

Indications

Acute ST segment elevation MI (STEMI) within 6 hours of symptom onset where primary percutaneous coronary intervention (PPCI) is **NOT** readily available.

Ensure patient fulfils the criteria for drug administration following the local protocols. Variation of these criteria is justifiable at local level with agreement of appropriate key stakeholders (e.g. cardiac network, or in the context of an approved clinical trial).

Contra-indications

Refer to local Trust checklist for thrombolytics.

Actions

Activates the fibrinolytic system, inducing the breaking up of intravascular thrombi and emboli.

Tenecteplase

TNK

Side Effects

Bleeding:

● Major – seek medical advice and transport to hospital rapidly.
● Minor e.g. at injection sites – use local pressure.

Arrhythmias – these are usually benign in the form of transient idioventricular rhythms and usually require no special treatment. Treat ventricular fibrillation (VF) as a complication of myocardial infarction (MI) with standard protocols; bradycardia with atropine as required.

Anaphylaxis – extremely rare (0.1%) with third generation bolus agents.

Hypotension – often responds to laying the patient flat.

Additional Information

PPCI is now the dominant reperfusion treatment and should be used where available; patients with STEMI will be taken direct to a specialist cardiac centre instead of receiving thrombolysis (**refer to acute coronary syndrome guideline**). Local protocol should be followed.

'Time is muscle!' Do not delay transportation to hospital if difficulties arise whilst setting up the equipment or establishing IV access. Qualified single responders should administer a thrombolytic if indicated while awaiting arrival of an ambulance.

Tenecteplase

TNK

In All Cases

Ensure a defibrillator is immediately available at all times.

Monitor conscious level, pulse, blood pressure and cardiac rhythm during and following injections. Manage complications (associated with the acute MI) as they occur using standard protocols. The main early adverse event associated with thrombolysis is bleeding, which should be managed according to standard protocols.

AT HOSPITAL – emphasise the need to commence a heparin infusion in accordance with local protocols – to reduce the risk of re-infarction.

Thrombolysis Checklist

Is primary PCI available?
- **YES** – undertake a **TIME CRITICAL** transfer to PPCI capable hospital.
- **NO** – refer to local Trust checklists for thrombolytics.

Tenecteplase   **TNK**

Dosage and Administration

1. Administer a bolus of intravenous injection of un-fractionated heparin before administration of tenecteplase (**refer to heparin guideline**). Flush the cannula well with saline.

2. **AT HOSPITAL** – It is essential that the care of the patient is handed over as soon as possible to a member of hospital staff qualified to administer a heparin infusion.

Route: Intravenous single bolus adjusted for patient weight.

AGE	WEIGHT DOSE	INITIAL DOSE	REPEAT DOSE	DOSE INTERVAL	VOLUME	MAXIMUM DOSE
≥18 years 1,000 U/ml	<60 kg (<9st 6lbs)	6000 units	NONE	N/A	6 ml	6,000 units
≥18 years 1,000 U/ml	60–69 kg (9st 6lbs – 10st 13lbs)	7000 units	NONE	N/A	7 ml	7,000 units
≥18 years 1,000 U/ml	70–79 kg (11st – 12st 7lbs)	8000 units	NONE	N/A	8 ml	8,000 units
≥18 years 1,000 U/ml	80–90 kg (12st 8lbs – 14st 2lbs)	9000 units	NONE	N/A	9 ml	9,000 units
≥18 years 1,000 U/ml	>90 kg (>14st 2lbs)	10,000 units	NONE	N/A	10 ml	10,000 units

Tetracaine 4%

Presentation

1 or 1.5 gram tubes of white semi-transparent gel.

Transparent occlusive dressing.

Indications

Where venepuncture may be required in a non-urgent situation, in individuals who are believed to have a fear of, or likely to become upset if undergoing venepuncture (usually children, some vulnerable adults or needle-phobic adults). Venepuncture includes intravenous injection, cannulation and obtaining venous blood.

Time of application should be noted and included in hand-over to the emergency department or other care facility.

Actions

Tetracaine 4% cream is a local anaesthetic agent, that has properties that allow it to penetrate intact skin, thus providing local anaesthesia to the area of skin with which it has been in contact.

Contra-indications

DO NOT apply tetracaine in the following circumstances:

- The application of tetracaine should not take preference over life-saving or any other clinically urgent procedures.
- If the area being considered for anaesthesia will require venepuncture in less than 15 minutes.
- Known allergy to tetracaine cream, or any of its other constituents.
- Known allergy to the brand of transparent occlusive dressing.

Tetracaine 4% TTC

- If the patient is allergic to other local anaesthetics.
- If the patient is pregnant or breastfeeding.
- If the patient is less than one month old.
- Avoid applying to open wounds, broken skin, lips, mouth, eyes, ears, anal, or genital region, mucous membranes.

Cautions

Allergy to Elastoplast or other adhesive dressing – discuss risk/benefit with carer.

Side Effects

Expect mild vasodilatation over the treated area.

Occasionally local irritation may occur.

Additional Information

Although the application of tetracaine may not directly improve the quality of care experienced by the patient from the ambulance service, it is in line with good patient care, and its use will benefit the patient's subsequent management.

Tetracaine takes 30–40 minutes after application before the area will become numb and remain numb for 4–6 hours.

Sites of application should be based on local guidelines.

Tetracaine 4%

TTC

Tetracaine only needs refrigeration if it is unlikely to be used for a considerable time; therefore bulk stores should be kept refrigerated. Generally speaking, it does not require refrigeration in everyday use, however tubes that are not refrigerated or used within 3 months should be discarded.

Special Precautions

Do not leave on for more than an hour.

Do not delay transfer to further care of TIME CRITICAL patients.

Dosage and Administration

- Apply one tube directly over a vein that looks as if it would support cannulation – refer to local care guideline.
- Do not rub the cream in.
- Place an occlusive dressing directly over the 'blob' of cream, taking care to completely surround the cream to ensure it does not leak out.
- Repeat the procedure in one similar, alternative site.
- **REMEMBER** to tell the receiving staff the time of application and location when handing the patient over.

Route: Topical.

AGE	INITIAL DOSE	REPEAT DOSE	DOSE INTERVAL	VOLUME	MAXIMUM DOSE
>1 month 4%	1–1.5 grams	N/A	N/A	1 tube	N/A

Tranexamic Acid   TXA

Presentation

Vial containing 500 mg tranexamic acid in 5 ml (100 mg/ml).

Indications

- Patients with **TIME CRITICAL** injury where significant internal/external haemorrhage is suspected.
- Injured patients fulfilling local Step 1 or Step 2 trauma triage protocol.

Actions

Tranexamic acid is an anti-fibrinolytic which reduces the breakdown of blood clot.

Contra-indications

- Isolated head injury.
- Critical interventions required (if critical interventions leave insufficient time for TXA administration).
- Bleeding now stopped.

Side Effects

Rapid injection might rarely cause hypotension.

Additional Information

- There is good data that this treatment is safe and effective (giving a 9% reduction in the number of deaths in patients in the CRASH2 trial).

Tranexamic Acid

TXA

- There is no evidence about whether or not tranexamic acid is effective in patients with head injury; however there is no evidence of harm.
- High dose regimes have been associated with convulsions; however, in the low dose regime recommended here, the benefit from giving TXA in trauma outweighs the risk of convulsions.

Dosage and Administration

Route: Intravenous only – **administer SLOWLY over 10 minutes – can be given as 10 aliquots administered 1 minute apart**.

AGE	INITIAL DOSE	REPEAT DOSE	DOSE INTERVAL	VOLUME	MAXIMUM DOSE
>12 years – adult 100 mg/ml	1 gram	NONE	N/A	10 mls	1 gram

PAGE FOR AGE

Page for Age

BIRTH

Vital Signs

GUIDE WEIGHT 3.5 kg	HEART RATE 110–160	RESPIRATION RATE 30–40	SYSTOLIC BLOOD PRESSURE 70–90

Airway Size by Type

OROPHARYNGEAL AIRWAY	LARYNGEAL MASK	I-GEL AIRWAY	ENDOTRACHEAL TUBE
000	1	1	Diameter: **3 mm**; Length: **10 cm**

Defibrillation – Cardiac Arrest

MANUAL	AUTOMATED EXTERNAL DEFIBRILLATOR
20 Joules	Where possible, use a manual defibrillator. If an AED is the only defibrillator available, it should be used (preferably using paediatric attenuation pads or else in paediatric mode).

Intravascular Fluid

FLUID	INITIAL DOSE	REPEAT DOSE	DOSE INTERVAL	VOLUME	MAXIMUM DOSE
Sodium chloride (5 ml/kg) 0.9% (IV/IO)	20 ml	20 ml	PRN	20 ml	140 ml
Sodium chloride (10 ml/kg) 0.9% (IV/IO)	35 ml	35 ml	PRN	35 ml	140 ml
Sodium chloride (20 ml/kg) 0.9% (IV/IO)	70 ml	70 ml	PRN	70 ml	140 ml

Cardiac Arrest

DRUG	INITIAL DOSE	REPEAT DOSE	DOSE INTERVAL	VOLUME	MAXIMUM DOSE
ADRENALINE (IV/IO) 1 milligram in 10 ml (1:10,000)	35 micrograms	35 micrograms	3–5 mins	0.35 ml	No limit
AMIODARONE (IV/IO) 300 milligrams in 10 ml	18 milligrams (after 3rd shock)	18 milligrams	After 5th shock	0.6 ml	36 milligrams
ATROPINE* (IV/IO) 100 micrograms in 1 ml	100 micrograms	NONE	N/A	1 ml	100 micrograms
ATROPINE* (IV/IO) 200 micrograms in 1 ml	100 micrograms	NONE	N/A	0.5 ml	100 micrograms
ATROPINE* (IV/IO) 300 micrograms in 1 ml	100 micrograms	NONE	N/A	0.3 ml	100 micrograms
ATROPINE* (IV/IO) 600 micrograms in 1 ml	100 micrograms	NONE	N/A	0.17 ml	100 micrograms

BRADYCARDIA in children is most commonly caused by **HYPOXIA**, requiring immediate **ABC** care. **NOT** drug therapy; therefore **ONLY** administer atropine in cases of bradycardia caused by vagal stimulation (e.g. suction).

Reversal of respiratory and central nervous system depression in a neonate following maternal opioid use during labour – single dose only

BIRTH Page for Age

DRUG	INITIAL DOSE	REPEAT DOSE	DOSE INTERVAL	VOLUME	MAXIMUM DOSE
Naloxone* (IM) 400 micrograms in 1 ml NB cautions	200 micrograms	NONE	N/A	0.5 ml	200 micrograms

*Reversal of respiratory arrest/extreme respiratory depression.

DRUG	INITIAL DOSE	REPEAT DOSE	DOSE INTERVAL	VOLUME	MAXIMUM DOSE
ADRENALINE (IM) anaphylaxis/asthma 1 milligram in 1 ml (1:1,000)	150 micrograms	150 micrograms	5 minutes	0.15 ml	No limit
BENZYLPENICILLIN (IV/IO) 600 milligrams in 9.6 ml	300 milligrams	NONE	N/A	5 ml	300 milligrams
BENZYLPENICILLIN (IM) 600 milligrams in 1.6 ml	300 milligrams	NONE	N/A	1 ml	300 milligrams
CHLORPHENAMINE (Oral)	N/A	N/A	N/A	N/A	N/A
CHLORPHENAMINE (IV/IO)	N/A	N/A	N/A	N/A	N/A
DEXAMETHASONE – croup (Oral)	N/A	N/A	N/A	N/A	N/A
DIAZEPAM (IV/IO) 10 milligrams in 2 ml	1 milligram	NONE	N/A	0.2 ml	1 milligram
DIAZEPAM (PR) 2.5 milligrams in 1.25 ml	1.25 or 2.5 milligrams	NONE	N/A	½ × 2.5 milligram tube or 1 × 2.5 milligram tube	1.25 or 2.5 milligrams

BIRTH Page for Age

Drug Therapy

DRUG	INITIAL DOSE	REPEAT DOSE	DOSE INTERVAL	VOLUME	MAXIMUM DOSE
GLUCAGON (IM) 1 milligram per vial	100 micrograms	NONE	N/A	0.1 vial	100 micrograms
GLUCOSE 10% (IV/IO) 50 grams in 500 ml	900 milligrams	900 milligrams	5 minutes	9 ml	2.7 grams
HYDROCORTISONE (IV/IO/IM) 100 milligrams in 1 ml	10 milligrams	NONE	N/A	0.1 ml	10 milligrams
HYDROCORTISONE (IV/IO/IM) 100 milligrams in 2 ml	10 milligrams	NONE	N/A	0.2 ml	10 milligrams
IBUPROFEN (Oral)	N/A	N/A	N/A	N/A	N/A
IPRATROPIUM (Neb)	N/A	N/A	N/A	N/A	N/A
PATIENT'S OWN MIDAZOLAM* (Buccal) 10 milligrams in 1 ml	1 milligram	NONE	N/A	0.1 ml	1 milligram
MORPHINE (IV/IO)	N/A	N/A	N/A	N/A	N/A
MORPHINE (Oral)	N/A	NONE	N/A	N/A	N/A

*Give the dose as prescribed in the child's individualised treatment plan (the dosages described above reflect the recommended dosages for a child of this age).

BIRTH Page for Age

DRUG	INITIAL DOSE	REPEAT DOSE	DOSE INTERVAL	VOLUME	MAXIMUM DOSE
NALOXONE**† (IV/IO) NB cautions 400 micrograms in 1 ml	40 micrograms	40 micrograms	3 minutes	0.1 ml	440 micrograms
NALOXONE** – INITIAL DOSE (IM) 400 micrograms in 1 ml	40 micrograms	See below	3 minutes	0.1 ml	See below
NALOXONE** – REPEAT DOSE (IM) 400 micrograms in 1 ml	–	400 micrograms	–	1 ml	440 micrograms
ONDANSETRON (Oral)	N/A	N/A	N/A	N/A	N/A
PARACETAMOL (Oral)	N/A	N/A	N/A	N/A	N/A
PARACETAMOL (IV/IO)	N/A	N/A	N/A	N/A	N/A
SALBUTAMOL (Neb)	N/A	N/A	N/A	N/A	N/A
TRANEXAMIC ACID (IV) 100 mg/ml	50 mg	NONE	N/A	0.5 ml	50 mg

*Reversal of respiratory and central nervous system depression in a neonate following maternal opioid use during labour – single dose only.

Intramuscular naloxone is used to reverse respiratory and central nervous system depression in a neonate following maternal opioid use during labour. For this specific indication, the dose is described in a separate box on page 214.

1 MONTH

Page for Age

Vital Signs

GUIDE WEIGHT 4.5 kg	HEART RATE 110–160	RESPIRATION RATE 30–40	SYSTOLIC BLOOD PRESSURE 70–90

Airway Size by Type

OROPHARYNGEAL AIRWAY	LARYNGEAL MASK	I-GEL AIRWAY	ENDOTRACHEAL TUBE
00	1	1	Diameter: **3 mm**; Length: **10 cm**

Defibrillation – Cardiac Arrest

MANUAL	AUTOMATED EXTERNAL DEFIBRILLATOR
20 Joules	Where possible, use a manual defibrillator. If an AED is the only defibrillator available, it should be used (preferably using paediatric attenuation pads or else in paediatric mode).

Intravascular Fluid

FLUID	INITIAL DOSE	REPEAT DOSE	DOSE INTERVAL	VOLUME	MAXIMUM DOSE
Sodium chloride (5 ml/kg) (IV/IO) 0.9%	20 ml	20 ml	PRN	20 ml	180 ml
Sodium chloride (10 ml/kg) (IV/IO) 0.9%	45 ml	45 ml	PRN	45 ml	180 ml
Sodium chloride (20 ml/kg) (IV/IO) 0.9%	90 ml	90 ml	PRN	90 ml	180 ml

1 MONTH Page for Age

DRUG	INITIAL DOSE	REPEAT DOSE	DOSE INTERVAL	VOLUME	MAXIMUM DOSE
ADRENALINE (IV/IO) 1 milligram in 10 ml (1:10,000)	50 micrograms	50 micrograms	3–5 mins	0.5 ml	No limit
AMIODARONE (IV/IO) 300 milligrams in 10 ml	25 milligrams (after 3rd shock)	25 milligrams	After 5th shock	0.8 ml	50 milligrams
ATROPINE* (IV/IO) 100 micrograms in 1 ml	100 micrograms	NONE	N/A	1 ml	100 micrograms
ATROPINE* (IV/IO) 200 micrograms in 1 ml	100 micrograms	NONE	N/A	0.5 ml	100 micrograms
ATROPINE* (IV/IO) 300 micrograms in 1 ml	100 micrograms	NONE	N/A	0.3 ml	100 micrograms
ATROPINE* (IV/IO) 600 micrograms in 1 ml	100 micrograms	NONE	N/A	0.17 ml	100 micrograms

BRADYCARDIA in children is most commonly caused by **HYPOXIA**, requiring immediate **ABC** care, **NOT** drug therapy; therefore **ONLY** administer atropine in cases of bradycardia caused by vagal stimulation (e.g. suction).

Drug Therapy

DRUG	INITIAL DOSE	REPEAT DOSE	DOSE INTERVAL	VOLUME	MAXIMUM DOSE
ADRENALINE (IM) anaphylaxis/asthma 1 milligram in 1 ml (1:1,000)	150 micrograms	150 micrograms	5 minutes	0.15 ml	No limit
BENZYLPENICILLIN (IV/IO) 600 milligrams in 9.6 ml	300 milligrams	NONE	N/A	5 ml	300 milligrams
BENZYLPENICILLIN (IM) 600 milligrams in 1.6 ml	300 milligrams	NONE	N/A	1 ml	300 milligrams
CHLORPHENAMINE (Oral)	N/A	N/A	N/A	N/A	N/A
CHLORPHENAMINE (IV/IO)	N/A	N/A	N/A	N/A	N/A
DEXAMETHASONE – croup (Oral) 3.8 milligrams per ml (use intravenous preparation orally)	1.9 milligrams	NONE	N/A	0.5 ml	1.9 milligrams
DIAZEPAM (IV/IO) 10 milligrams in 2 ml	1.5 milligrams	NONE	N/A	0.3 ml	1.5 milligrams
DIAZEPAM (PR) 5 milligrams in 2.5 ml	5 milligrams	NONE	N/A	1 × 5 milligram tube	5 milligrams

1 MONTH Page for Age

DRUG	INITIAL DOSE	REPEAT DOSE	DOSE INTERVAL	VOLUME	MAXIMUM DOSE
GLUCAGON (IM) 1 milligram per vial	500 micrograms	NONE	N/A	0.5 vial	500 micrograms
GLUCOSE 10% (IV/IO) 50 grams in 500 ml	1 gram	1 gram	5 minutes	10 ml	5 grams
HYDROCORTISONE (IV/IO/IM) 100 milligrams in 1 ml	25 milligrams	NONE	N/A	0.25 ml	25 milligrams
HYDROCORTISONE (IV/IO/IM) 100 milligrams in 1 ml	25 milligrams	NONE	N/A	0.25 ml	25 milligrams
IBUPROFEN (Oral) 100 milligrams in 2 ml	N/A	N/A	N/A	0.5 ml	25 milligrams
IPRATROPIUM (Neb) 250 micrograms in 1 ml	125 – 250 micrograms	NONE	N/A	0.5 ml – 1 ml	125 – 250 micrograms
IPRATROPIUM (Neb) 500 micrograms in 2 ml	125 – 250 micrograms	NONE	N/A	0.5 ml – 1 ml	125 – 250 micrograms
MIDAZOLAM* (Buccal) 10 milligrams in 1 ml	1.5 milligrams	NONE	N/A	0.15 ml	1.5 milligrams
PATIENT'S OWN					
IPRATROPIUM (IV/IO)	N/A	N/A	N/A	N/A	125 – 250 micrograms
MORPHINE (Oral)	N/A	N/A	N/A	N/A	N/A
MORPHINE (IV/IO)	N/A	N/A	N/A	N/A	N/A
NALOXONE (IV/IO) 400 micrograms in 1 ml	40 micrograms	40 micrograms	3 minutes	0.1 ml	440 micrograms
NALOXONE NB cautions					

Give the dose as prescribed in the child's individualised treatment plan (the dosages described above reflect the recommended dosages for a child of this age).

DRUG	INITIAL DOSE	REPEAT DOSE	DOSE INTERVAL	VOLUME	MAXIMUM DOSE
NALOXONE – INITIAL DOSE (IM) 400 micrograms in 1 ml	40 micrograms	See below	3 minutes	0.1 ml	See below
NALOXONE – REPEAT DOSE (IM) 400 micrograms in 1 ml	–	400 micrograms	–	1 ml	440 micrograms
ONDANSETRON (IV/IO/IM) 2 milligrams in 1 ml	0.5 milligrams	NONE	N/A	0.25 ml	0.5 milligrams
PARACETAMOL (Oral)	N/A	N/A	N/A	N/A	N/A
PARACETAMOL (IV/IO)	N/A	N/A	N/A	N/A	N/A
SALBUTAMOL (Neb) 2.5 milligrams in 2.5 ml	2.5 milligrams	2.5 milligrams	5 minutes	2.5 ml	N/A
SALBUTAMOL (Neb) 5 milligrams in 2.5 ml	2.5 milligrams	2.5 milligrams	5 minutes	1.25 ml	N/A
TRANEXAMIC ACID (IV) 100 mg/ml	50 mg	NONE	N/A	0.5 ml	50 mg

This page left intentionally blank for your notes

Page for Age

3 MONTHS

Vital Signs

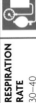 GUIDE WEIGHT 6 kg	HEART RATE 110–160	RESPIRATION RATE 30–40	SYSTOLIC BLOOD PRESSURE 70–90

Airway Size by Type

OROPHARYNGEAL AIRWAY	LARYNGEAL MASK	I-GEL AIRWAY	ENDOTRACHEAL TUBE
00	1.5	1.5	Diameter: **3.5 mm**; Length: **11 cm**

Defibrillation – Cardiac Arrest

MANUAL	AUTOMATED EXTERNAL DEFIBRILLATOR
25 Joules	Where possible, use a manual defibrillator. If an AED is the only defibrillator available, it should be used (preferably using paediatric attenuation pads or else in paediatric mode).

Intravascular Fluid

FLUID	INITIAL DOSE	REPEAT DOSE	DOSE INTERVAL	VOLUME	MAXIMUM DOSE
Sodium chloride (5 ml/kg) (IV/IO) 0.9%	30 ml	30 ml	PRN	30 ml	240 ml
Sodium chloride (10 ml/kg) (IV/IO) 0.9%	60 ml	60 ml	PRN	60 ml	240 ml
Sodium chloride (20 ml/kg) (IV/IO) 0.9%	120 ml	120 ml	PRN	120 ml	240 ml

DRUG	INITIAL DOSE	REPEAT DOSE	DOSE INTERVAL	VOLUME	MAXIMUM DOSE
ADRENALINE (IV/IO) 1 milligram in 10 ml (1:10,000)	60 micrograms	60 micrograms	3–5 mins	0.6 ml	No limit
AMIODARONE (IV/IO) 300 milligrams in 10 ml	30 milligrams (after 3rd shock)	30 milligrams	After 5th shock	1 ml	60 milligrams
ATROPINE* (IV/IO) 100 micrograms in 1 ml	120 micrograms	NONE	N/A	1.2 ml	120 micrograms
ATROPINE* (IV/IO) 200 micrograms in 1 ml	120 micrograms	NONE	N/A	0.6 ml	120 micrograms
ATROPINE* (IV/IO) 300 micrograms in 1 ml	120 micrograms	NONE	N/A	0.4 ml	120 micrograms
ATROPINE* (IV/IO) 600 micrograms in 1 ml	120 micrograms	NONE	N/A	0.2 ml	120 micrograms

BRADYCARDIA in children is most commonly caused by **HYPOXIA**, requiring immediate **ABC** care, **NOT** drug therapy; therefore **ONLY** administer atropine in cases of bradycardia caused by vagal stimulation (e.g. ...action).

Drug Therapy

3 MONTHS Page for Age

DRUG	INITIAL DOSE	REPEAT DOSE	DOSE INTERVAL	VOLUME	MAXIMUM DOSE
ADRENALINE (IM) anaphylaxis/asthma 1 milligram in 1 ml (1:1,000)	150 micrograms	150 micrograms	5 minutes	0.15 ml	No limit
BENZYLPENICILLIN (IV/IO) 600 milligrams in 9.6 ml	300 milligrams	NONE	N/A	5 ml	300 milligrams
BENZYLPENICILLIN (IM) 600 milligrams in 1.6 ml	300 milligrams	NONE	N/A	1 ml	300 milligrams
CHLORPHENAMINE (Oral)	N/A	N/A	N/A	N/A	N/A
CHLORPHENAMINE (IV/IO)	N/A	N/A	N/A	N/A	N/A
DEXAMETHASONE – croup (Oral) 3.8 milligrams per ml (use intravenous preparation orally)	1.9 milligrams	NONE	N/A	0.5 ml	1.9 milligrams
DIAZEPAM (IV/IO) 10 milligrams in 2 ml	2 milligrams	NONE	N/A	0.4 ml	2 milligrams
DIAZEPAM (PR) 5 milligrams in 2.5 ml	5 milligrams	NONE	N/A	1 × 5 milligram tube	5 milligrams

3 MONTHS Page for Age

DRUG	INITIAL DOSE	REPEAT DOSE	DOSE INTERVAL	VOLUME	MAXIMUM DOSE
GLUCAGON (IM) 1 milligram per vial	500 micrograms	NONE	N/A	0.5 vial	500 micrograms
GLUCOSE 10% (IV/IO) 50 grams in 500 ml	1 gram	1 gram	5 minutes	10 ml	3 grams
HYDROCORTISONE (IV/IO/IM) 100 milligrams in 1 ml	25 milligrams	NONE	N/A	0.25 ml	25 milligrams
HYDROCORTISONE (IV/IO/IM) 100 milligrams in 2 ml	25 milligrams	NONE	N/A	0.5 ml	25 milligrams
IBUPROFEN (Oral) 100 milligrams in 5 ml	50 milligrams	50 milligrams	8 hours	2.5 ml	150 milligrams
IPRATROPIUM (Neb) 100 micrograms in 1 ml	125 – 250 micrograms	NONE	N/A	0.5 ml – 1 ml	125 – 250 micrograms
IPRATROPIUM (Neb) 250 micrograms in 1 ml	125 – 250 micrograms	NONE	N/A	0.5 ml – 1 ml	125 – 250 micrograms
IPRATROPIUM (Neb) 500 micrograms in 2 ml	125 – 250 micrograms	NONE	N/A	0.5 ml – 1 ml	125 – 250 micrograms
PATIENT'S OWN MIDAZOLAM* (Buccal) 10 milligrams in 1 ml	2 milligrams	NONE	N/A	0.2 ml	2 milligrams
MORPHINE (IV/IO)	N/A	N/A	N/A	N/A	N/A
MORPHINE (Oral)	N/A	N/A	N/A	N/A	N/A

Give the dose as prescribed in the child's individualised treatment plan (the dosages described above reflect the recommended dosages for a child of this age).

Drug Therapy

DRUG	INITIAL DOSE	REPEAT DOSE	DOSE INTERVAL	VOLUME	MAXIMUM DOSE
NALOXONE (IV/IO) NB cautions 400 micrograms in 1 ml	60 micrograms	60 micrograms	3 minutes	0.15 ml	660 micrograms
NALOXONE – INITIAL DOSE (IM) 400 micrograms in 1 ml	60 micrograms	See below	3 minutes	0.15 ml	See below
NALOXONE – REPEAT DOSE (IM) 400 micrograms in 1 ml	–	400 micrograms	–	1 ml	460 micrograms
ONDANSETRON (IV/IO/IM) 2 milligrams in 1 ml	0.5 milligrams	NONE	N/A	0.25 ml	0.5 milligrams
PARACETAMOL (Oral) 120 milligrams in 5 ml – infant suspension	60 milligrams	60 milligrams	4–6 hours	2.5 ml	240 milligrams in 24 hours
PARACETAMOL (IV/IO)	N/A	N/A	N/A	N/A	N/A
SALBUTAMOL (Neb) 2.5 milligrams in 2.5 ml	2.5 milligrams	2.5 milligrams	5 minutes	2.5 ml	N/A
SALBUTAMOL (Neb) 5 milligrams in 2.5 ml	2.5 milligrams	2.5 milligrams	5 minutes	1.25 ml	N/A
TRANEXAMIC ACID (IV) 100 mg/ml	100 mg	NONE	N/A	1 ml	100 mg

This page left intentionally blank for your notes

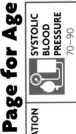

Page for Age

Vital Signs

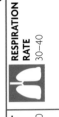 GUIDE WEIGHT 8 kg	HEART RATE 110–160	RESPIRATION RATE 30–40	SYSTOLIC BLOOD PRESSURE 70–90

6 MONTHS

Airway Size by Type

OROPHARYNGEAL AIRWAY	LARYNGEAL MASK	I-GEL AIRWAY	ENDOTRACHEAL TUBE
00	1.5	1.5	Diameter: **4 mm**; Length: **12 cm**

Defibrillation – Cardiac Arrest

MANUAL	AUTOMATED EXTERNAL DEFIBRILLATOR
40 Joules	Where possible, use a manual defibrillator. If an AED is the only defibrillator available, it should be used (preferably using paediatric attenuation pads or else in paediatric mode).

Intravascular Fluid

FLUID	INITIAL DOSE	REPEAT DOSE	DOSE INTERVAL	VOLUME	MAXIMUM DOSE
Sodium chloride (5 ml/kg) (IV/IO) 0.9%	40 ml	40 ml	PRN	40 ml	320 ml
Sodium chloride (10 ml/kg) (IV/IO) 0.9%	80 ml	80 ml	PRN	80 ml	320 ml
Sodium chloride (20 ml/kg) (IV/IO) 0.9%	160 ml	160 ml	PRN	160 ml	320 ml

6 MONTHS Page for Age

DRUG	INITIAL DOSE	REPEAT DOSE	DOSE INTERVAL	VOLUME	MAXIMUM DOSE
ADRENALINE (IV/IO) 1 milligram in 10 ml (1:10,000)	80 micrograms	80 micrograms	3–5 mins	0.8 ml	No limit
AMIODARONE (IV/IO) 300 milligrams in 10 ml	40 milligrams (after 3rd shock)	40 milligrams	After 5th shock	1.3 ml	80 milligrams
ATROPINE* (IV/IO) 100 micrograms in 1 ml	120 micrograms	NONE	N/A	1.2 ml	120 micrograms
ATROPINE* (IV/IO) 200 micrograms in 1 ml	120 micrograms	NONE	N/A	0.6 ml	120 micrograms
ATROPINE* (IV/IO) 300 micrograms in 1 ml	120 micrograms	NONE	N/A	0.4 ml	120 micrograms
ATROPINE* (IV/IO) 600 micrograms in 1 ml	120 micrograms	NONE	N/A	0.2 ml	120 micrograms

*BRADYCARDIA in children is most commonly caused by HYPOXIA, requiring immediate ABC care, NOT drug therapy; therefore ONLY administer atropine in cases of bradycardia caused by vagal stimulation (e.g. suction).

Drug Therapy

DRUG	INITIAL DOSE	REPEAT DOSE	DOSE INTERVAL	VOLUME	MAXIMUM DOSE
ADRENALINE (IM) anaphylaxis/asthma 1 milligram in 1 ml (1:1,000)	150 micrograms	150 micrograms	5 minutes	0.15 ml	No limit
BENZYLPENICILLIN (IV/IO) 600 milligrams in 9.6 ml	300 milligrams	NONE	N/A	5 ml	300 milligrams
BENZYLPENICILLIN (IM) 600 milligrams in 1.6 ml	300 milligrams	NONE	N/A	1 ml	300 milligrams
CHLORPHENAMINE (Oral)	N/A	N/A	N/A	N/A	N/A
CHLORPHENAMINE (IV/IO)	N/A	N/A	N/A	N/A	N/A
DEXAMETHASONE – croup (Oral) 3.8 milligrams per ml (use intravenous preparation orally)	1.9 milligrams	NONE	N/A	0.5 ml	1.9 milligrams
DIAZEPAM (IV/IO) 10 milligrams in 2 ml	2.5 milligrams	NONE	N/A	0.5 ml	2.5 milligrams
DIAZEPAM (PR) 5 milligrams in 2.5 ml	5 milligrams	NONE	N/A	1 × 5 milligram tube	5 milligrams

DRUG	INITIAL DOSE	REPEAT DOSE	DOSE INTERVAL	VOLUME	MAXIMUM DOSE
GLUCAGON (IM) 1 milligram per vial	500 micrograms	NONE	N/A	0.5 vial	500 micrograms
GLUCOSE 10% (IV/IO) 50 grams in 500 ml	1.5 grams	1.5 grams	5 minutes	15 ml	4.5 grams
HYDROCORTISONE (IV/IO/IM) 100 milligrams in 1 ml	50 milligrams	NONE	N/A	0.5 ml	50 milligrams
HYDROCORTISONE (IV/IO/IM) 100 milligrams in 2 ml	50 milligrams	NONE	N/A	1 ml	50 milligrams
IBUPROFEN (Oral) 100 milligrams in 5 ml	50 milligrams	50 milligrams	8 hours	2.5 ml	150 milligrams
IPRATROPIUM (Neb) 250 micrograms in 1 ml	125 – 250 micrograms	NONE	N/A	0.5 ml – 1 ml	125 – 250 micrograms
IPRATROPIUM (Neb) 500 micrograms in 2 ml	125 – 250 micrograms	NONE	N/A	0.5 ml – 1 ml	125 – 250 micrograms
PATIENT'S OWN MIDAZOLAM* (Buccal) 10 milligrams in 1 ml	2.5 milligrams	NONE	N/A	0.25 ml	2.5 milligrams
MORPHINE (IV/IO)	N/A	N/A	N/A	N/A	N/A
MORPHINE (Oral)	N/A	N/A	N/A	N/A	N/A

Give the dose as prescribed in the child's individualised treatment plan (the dosages described above reflect the recommended dosages for a child of this age).

DRUG	INITIAL DOSE	REPEAT DOSE	DOSE INTERVAL	VOLUME	MAXIMUM DOSE
NALOXONE (IV/IO) NB cautions 400 micrograms in 1 ml	80 micrograms	80 micrograms	3 minutes	0.2 ml	880 micrograms
NALOXONE **– INITIAL DOSE** (IM) 400 micrograms in 1 ml	80 micrograms	See below	3 minutes	0.2 ml	See below
NALOXONE **– REPEAT DOSE** (IM) 400 micrograms in 1 ml	–	400 micrograms	–	1 ml	480 micrograms
ONDANSETRON (IV/IO/IM) 2 milligrams in 1 ml	1 milligram	NONE	N/A	0.5 ml	1 milligram
PARACETAMOL (Oral) 120 milligrams in 5 ml – infant suspension	120 milligrams	120 milligrams	4 – 6 hours	5 ml	480 milligrams in 24 hours
PARACETAMOL (IV/IO) 10 milligrams in 1 ml	50 milligrams	50 milligrams	4 – 6 hours	5 ml	200 milligrams in 24 hours
SALBUTAMOL (Neb) 2.5 milligrams in 2.5 ml	2.5 milligrams	2.5 milligrams	5 minutes	2.5 ml	No limit
SALBUTAMOL (Neb) 5 milligrams in 2.5 ml	2.5 milligrams	2.5 milligrams	5 minutes	1.25 ml	No limit
TRANEXAMIC ACID (IV) 100 mg/ml	100 mg	NONE	N/A	1 ml	100 mg

This page left intentionally blank for your notes

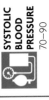

9 MONTHS

Page for Age

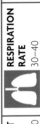 **Vital Signs**

GUIDE WEIGHT 9 kg	HEART RATE 110–160	RESPIRATION RATE 30–40	SYSTOLIC BLOOD PRESSURE 70–90

Airway Size by Type

OROPHARYNGEAL AIRWAY	LARYNGEAL MASK	I-GEL AIRWAY	ENDOTRACHEAL TUBE
00	1.5	1.5	Diameter: **4 mm**; Length: **12 cm**

Defibrillation – Cardiac Arrest

MANUAL	AUTOMATED EXTERNAL DEFIBRILLATOR
40 Joules	Where possible, use a manual defibrillator. If an AED is the only defibrillator available, it should be used (preferably using paediatric attenuation pads or else in paediatric mode).

Intravascular Fluid

FLUID	INITIAL DOSE	REPEAT DOSE	DOSE INTERVAL	VOLUME	MAXIMUM DOSE
Sodium chloride (5 ml/kg) 0.9% (IV/IO)	45 ml	45 ml	PRN	45 ml	360 ml
Sodium chloride (10 ml/kg) 0.9% (IV/IO)	90 ml	90 ml	PRN	90 ml	360 ml
Sodium chloride (20 ml/kg) 0.9% (IV/IO)	180 ml	180 ml	PRN	180 ml	360 ml

9 MONTHS Page for Age

DRUG	INITIAL DOSE	REPEAT DOSE	DOSE INTERVAL	VOLUME	MAXIMUM DOSE
ADRENALINE (IV/IO) 1 milligram in 10 ml (1:10,000)	90 micrograms	90 micrograms	3–5 mins	0.9 ml	No limit
AMIODARONE (IV/IO) 300 milligrams in 10 ml	45 milligrams (after 3rd shock)	45 milligrams	After 5th shock	1.5 ml	90 milligrams
ATROPINE* (IV/IO) 100 micrograms in 1 ml	120 micrograms	NONE	N/A	1.2 ml	120 micrograms
ATROPINE* (IV/IO) 200 micrograms in 1 ml	120 micrograms	NONE	N/A	0.6 ml	120 micrograms
ATROPINE* (IV/IO) 300 micrograms in 1 ml	120 micrograms	NONE	N/A	0.4 ml	120 micrograms
ATROPINE* (IV/IO) 600 micrograms in 1 ml	120 micrograms	NONE	N/A	0.2 ml	120 micrograms

*BRADYCARDIA in children is most commonly caused by HYPOXIA, requiring immediate ABC care, NOT drug therapy; therefore ONLY administer atropine in cases of bradycardia caused by vagal stimulation (e.g. suction).

Drug Therapy

DRUG	INITIAL DOSE	REPEAT DOSE	DOSE INTERVAL	VOLUME	MAXIMUM DOSE
ADRENALINE (IM) anaphylaxis/asthma 1 milligram in 1 ml (1:1,000)	150 micrograms	150 micrograms	5 minutes	0.15 ml	No limit
BENZYLPENICILLIN (IV/IO) 600 milligrams in 9.6 ml	300 milligrams	NONE	N/A	5 ml	300 milligrams
BENZYLPENICILLIN (IM) 600 milligrams in 1.6 ml	300 milligrams	NONE	N/A	1 ml	300 milligrams
CHLORPHENAMINE (Oral)	N/A	N/A	N/A	N/A	N/A
CHLORPHENAMINE (IV/IO)	N/A	N/A	N/A	N/A	N/A
DEXAMETHASONE – croup (Oral) 3.8 milligrams per ml (use intravenous preparation orally)	1.9 milligrams	NONE	N/A	0.5 ml	1.9 milligrams
DIAZEPAM (IV/IO) 10 milligrams in 2 ml	2.5 milligrams	NONE	N/A	0.5 ml	2.5 milligrams
DIAZEPAM (PR) 5 milligrams in 2.5 ml	5 milligrams	NONE	N/A	1 × 5 milligram tube	5 milligrams

9 MONTHS Page for Age

DRUG	INITIAL DOSE	REPEAT DOSE	DOSE INTERVAL	VOLUME	MAXIMUM DOSE
GLUCAGON (IM) 1 milligram per vial	500 micrograms	NONE	N/A	0.5 vial	500 micrograms
GLUCOSE 10% (IV/IO) 50 grams in 500 ml	2 grams	2 grams	5 minutes	20 ml	6 grams
HYDROCORTISONE (IV/IO/IM) 100 milligrams in 1 ml	50 milligrams	NONE	N/A	0.5 ml	50 milligrams
HYDROCORTISONE (IV/IO/IM) 100 milligrams in 2 ml	50 milligrams	NONE	N/A	1 ml	50 milligrams
IBUPROFEN (Oral) 100 milligrams in 5 ml	50 milligrams	50 milligrams	8 hours	2.5 ml	150 milligrams
IPRATROPIUM (Neb) 250 micrograms in 1 ml	125 – 250 micrograms	NONE	N/A	0.5 ml – 1 ml	125 – 250 micrograms
IPRATROPIUM (Neb) 500 micrograms in 2 ml	125 – 250 micrograms	NONE	N/A	0.5 ml – 1 ml	125 – 250 micrograms
MIDAZOLAM* (Buccal) 10 milligrams in 1 ml	2.5 milligrams	NONE	N/A	0.25 ml	2.5 milligrams
PATIENT'S OWN MORPHINE (IV/IO)	N/A	N/A	N/A	N/A	N/A
MORPHINE (Oral)	N/A	N/A	N/A	N/A	N/A

Give the dose as prescribed in the child's individualised treatment plan (the dosages described above reflect the recommended dosages for a child of this age).

Drug Therapy

DRUG	INITIAL DOSE	REPEAT DOSE	DOSE INTERVAL	VOLUME	MAXIMUM DOSE
NALOXONE (IV/IO) NB cautions 400 micrograms in 1 ml	80 micrograms	80 micrograms	3 minutes	0.2 ml	No limit
NALOXONE – INITIAL DOSE (IM) 400 micrograms in 1 ml	80 micrograms	See below	3 minutes	0.2 ml	See below
NALOXONE – REPEAT DOSE (IM) 400 micrograms in 1 ml	–	400 micrograms	–	1 ml	480 micrograms
ONDANSETRON (IV/IO/IM) 2 milligrams/ml	1 milligram	NONE	N/A	0.5 ml	1 milligram
PARACETAMOL (Oral) 120 milligrams in 5 ml – infant suspension	120 milligrams	120 milligrams	4 – 6 hours	5 ml	480 milligrams in 24 hours
PARACETAMOL (IV/IO) 10 milligrams in 1 ml	50 milligrams	50 milligrams	4 – 6 hours	5 ml	200 milligrams in 24 hours
SALBUTAMOL (Neb) 2.5 milligrams in 2.5 ml	2.5 milligrams	2.5 milligrams	5 minutes	2.5 ml	No limit
SALBUTAMOL (Neb) 5 milligrams in 2.5 ml	2.5 milligrams	2.5 milligrams	5 minutes	1.25 ml	No limit
TRANEXAMIC ACID (IV) 100 mg/ml	150 mg	NONE	N/A	1.5 ml	150 mg

This page left intentionally blank for your notes

Page for Age

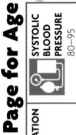

12 MONTHS

Vital Signs

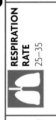 GUIDE WEIGHT 10 kg	HEART RATE 110–150	RESPIRATION RATE 25–35	SYSTOLIC BLOOD PRESSURE 80–95

Airway Size by Type

OROPHARYNGEAL AIRWAY	LARYNGEAL MASK	I-GEL AIRWAY	ENDOTRACHEAL TUBE
00 OR 0	1.5	1.5 OR 2	Diameter: **4.5 mm**; Length: **13 cm**

Defibrillation – Cardiac Arrest

MANUAL	AUTOMATED EXTERNAL DEFIBRILLATOR
40 Joules	A standard AED (either with paediatric attenuation pads or else in paediatric mode) can be used. If paediatric pads are not available, standard adult pads can be used (but must not overlap).

Intravascular Fluid

FLUID	INITIAL DOSE	REPEAT DOSE	DOSE INTERVAL	VOLUME	MAXIMUM DOSE
Sodium chloride (5 ml/kg) (IV/IO) 0.9%	50 ml	50 ml	PRN	50 ml	400 ml
Sodium chloride (10 ml/kg) (IV/IO) 0.9%	100 ml	100 ml	PRN	100 ml	400 ml
Sodium chloride (20 ml/kg) (IV/IO) 0.9%	200 ml	200 ml	PRN	200 ml	400 ml

12 MONTHS Page for Age

DRUG	INITIAL DOSE	REPEAT DOSE	DOSE INTERVAL	VOLUME	MAXIMUM DOSE
ADRENALINE (IV/IO) 1 milligram in 10 ml (1:10,000)	100 micrograms	100 micrograms	3–5 mins	1 ml	No limit
AMIODARONE (IV/IO) 300 milligrams in 10 ml	50 milligrams (after 3rd shock)	50 milligrams	After 5th shock	1.7 ml	100 milligrams
ATROPINE* (IV/IO) 100 micrograms in 1 ml	200 micrograms	NONE	N/A	2ml	200 micrograms
ATROPINE* (IV/IO) 200 micrograms in 1 ml	200 micrograms	NONE	N/A	1 ml	200 micrograms
ATROPINE* (IV/IO) 300 micrograms in 1 ml	200 micrograms	NONE	N/A	0.7 ml	200 micrograms
ATROPINE* (IV/IO) 600 micrograms in 1 ml	200 micrograms	NONE	N/A	0.3 ml	200 micrograms

*BRADYCARDIA in children is most commonly caused by HYPOXIA, requiring immediate ABC care, NOT drug therapy; therefore ONLY administer atropine in cases of bradycardia caused by vagal stimulation (e.g. suction).

DRUG	INITIAL DOSE	REPEAT DOSE	DOSE INTERVAL	VOLUME	MAXIMUM DOSE
ADRENALINE (IM) anaphylaxis/asthma 1 milligram in 1 ml (1:1,000)	150 micrograms	150 micrograms	5 minutes	0.15 ml	No limit
BENZYLPENICILLIN (IV/IO) 600 milligrams in 9.6 ml	600 milligrams	NONE	N/A	10 ml	600 milligrams
BENZYLPENICILLIN (IM) 600 milligrams in 1.6 ml	600 milligrams	NONE	N/A	2 ml	600 milligrams
CHLORPHENAMINE (Oral) Various	1 milligram	NONE	N/A	N/A	N/A
CHLORPHENAMINE (IV/IO/IM) 10 milligrams in 1 ml	2.5 milligrams	NONE	N/A	0.25 ml	2.5 milligrams
DEXAMETHASONE – croup (Oral) 3.8 milligrams per ml (use intravenous preparation orally)	1.9 milligrams	NONE	N/A	0.5 ml	1.9 milligrams
DIAZEPAM (IV/IO) 10 milligrams in 2 ml	3 milligrams	NONE	N/A	0.6 ml	3 milligrams
DIAZEPAM (PR) 5 milligrams in 2.5 ml	5 milligrams	NONE	N/A	1 × 5 milligram tube	5 milligrams

Drug Therapy

DRUG	INITIAL DOSE	REPEAT DOSE	DOSE INTERVAL	VOLUME	MAXIMUM DOSE
GLUCAGON (IM) 1 milligram per vial	500 micrograms	NONE	N/A	0.5 vial	500 micrograms
GLUCOSE 10% (IV/IO) 50 grams in 500 ml	2 grams	2 grams	5 minutes	20 ml	6 grams
HYDROCORTISONE (IV/IO/IM) 100 milligrams in 1 ml	50 milligrams	NONE	N/A	0.5 ml	50 milligrams
HYDROCORTISONE (IV/IO/IM) 100 milligrams in 2 ml	50 milligrams	NONE	N/A	1 ml	50 milligrams
IBUPROFEN (Oral) 100 milligrams in 5 ml	100 milligrams	100 milligrams	8 hours	5 ml	300 milligrams
IPRATROPIUM (Neb) 250 micrograms in 1 ml	125 – 250 micrograms	NONE	N/A	0.5 ml – 1 ml	125 – 250 micrograms
IPRATROPIUM (Neb) 500 micrograms in 2 ml	125 – 250 micrograms	NONE	N/A	0.5 ml – 1 ml	125 – 250 micrograms
PATIENT'S OWN **MIDAZOLAM*** (Buccal) 10 milligrams in 1 ml	5 milligrams	NONE	N/A	0.5 ml	5 milligrams
MORPHINE (IV/IO) 10 milligrams in 10 ml	1 milligram	1 milligram	5 minutes	1 ml	2 milligrams
MORPHINE (Oral) 10 milligrams in 5 ml	2 milligrams	NONE	N/A	1 ml	2 milligrams

*Give the dose as prescribed in the child's individualised treatment plan (the dosages described above reflect the recommended dosages for a child of this age).

Drug Therapy

12 MONTHS Page for Age

DRUG	INITIAL DOSE	REPEAT DOSE	DOSE INTERVAL	VOLUME	MAXIMUM DOSE
NALOXONE (IV/IO) NB cautions 400 micrograms in 1 ml	100 micrograms	100 micrograms	3 minutes	0.25 ml	No limit
NALOXONE – INITIAL DOSE (IM) 400 micrograms in 1 ml	100 micrograms	See below	3 minutes	0.25 ml	See below
NALOXONE – REPEAT DOSE (IM) 400 micrograms in 1 ml	–	400 micrograms	–	1 ml	500 micrograms
ONDANSETRON (IV/IO/IM) 2 milligrams in 1 ml	1 milligram	NONE	N/A	0.5 ml	1 milligram
PARACETAMOL (Oral) 120 milligrams in 5 ml – infant suspension	120 milligrams	120 milligrams	4 – 6 hours	5 ml	480 milligrams in 24 hours
PARACETAMOL (IV/IO) 10 milligrams in 1 ml	125 milligrams	125 milligrams	4 – 6 hours	12.5 ml	500 milligrams in 24 hours
SALBUTAMOL (Neb) 2.5 milligrams in 2.5 ml	2.5 milligrams	2.5 milligrams	5 minutes	2.5 ml	No limit
SALBUTAMOL (Neb) 5 milligrams in 2.5 ml	2.5 milligrams	2.5 milligrams	5 minutes	1.25 ml	No limit
TRANEXAMIC ACID (IV) 100 mg/ml	150 mg	NONE	N/A	1.5 ml	150 mg

This page left intentionally blank for your notes

Page for Age

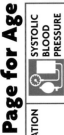

18 MONTHS

Vital Signs

GUIDE WEIGHT	HEART RATE	RESPIRATION RATE	SYSTOLIC BLOOD PRESSURE
11 kg	110–150	25–35	80–95

Airway Size by Type

OROPHARYNGEAL AIRWAY	LARYNGEAL MASK	I-GEL AIRWAY	ENDOTRACHEAL TUBE
00 OR 0	2	1.5 OR 2	Diameter: **4.5 mm**; Length: **13 cm**

Defibrillation – Cardiac Arrest

MANUAL	AUTOMATED EXTERNAL DEFIBRILLATOR
50 Joules	A standard AED (either with paediatric attenuation pads or else in paediatric mode) can be used. If paediatric pads are not available, standard adult pads can be used (but must not overlap).

Intravascular Fluid

FLUID	INITIAL DOSE	REPEAT DOSE	DOSE INTERVAL	VOLUME	MAXIMUM DOSE
Sodium chloride (5 ml/kg) (IV/IO) 0.9%	55 ml	55 ml	PRN	55 ml	440 ml
Sodium chloride (10 ml/kg) (IV/IO) 0.9%	110 ml	110 ml	PRN	110 ml	440 ml
Sodium chloride (20 ml/kg) (IV/IO) 0.9%	220 ml	220 ml	PRN	220 ml	440 ml

18 MONTHS Page for Age

DRUG	INITIAL DOSE	REPEAT DOSE	DOSE INTERVAL	VOLUME	MAXIMUM DOSE
ADRENALINE (IV/IO) 1 milligram in 10 ml (1:10,000)	110 micrograms	110 micrograms	3–5 mins	1.1 ml	No limit
AMIODARONE (IV/IO) 300 milligrams in 10 ml	55 milligrams (after 3rd shock)	55 milligrams	After 5th shock	1.8 ml	110 milligrams
ATROPINE* (IV/IO) 100 micrograms in 1 ml	200 micrograms	NONE	N/A	2 ml	200 micrograms
ATROPINE* (IV/IO) 200 micrograms in 1 ml	200 micrograms	NONE	N/A	1 ml	200 micrograms
ATROPINE* (IV/IO) 300 micrograms in 1 ml	200 micrograms	NONE	N/A	0.7 ml	200 micrograms
ATROPINE* (IV/IO) 600 micrograms in 1 ml	200 micrograms	NONE	N/A	0.3 ml	200 micrograms

*BRADYCARDIA in children is most commonly caused by **HYPOXIA**, requiring immediate **ABC** care, **NOT** drug therapy; therefore **ONLY** administer atropine in cases of bradycardia caused by vagal stimulation (e.g. suction).

Drug Therapy

DRUG	INITIAL DOSE	REPEAT DOSE	DOSE INTERVAL	VOLUME	MAXIMUM DOSE
ADRENALINE (IM) anaphylaxis/asthma 1 milligram in 1 ml (1:1,000)	150 micrograms	150 micrograms	5 minutes	0.15 ml	No limit
BENZYLPENICILLIN (IV/IO) 600 milligrams in 9.6 ml	600 milligrams	NONE	N/A	10 ml	600 milligrams
BENZYLPENICILLIN (IM) 600 milligrams in 1.6 ml	600 milligrams	NONE	N/A	2 ml	600 milligrams
CHLORPHENAMINE (Oral) Various	1 milligram	NONE	N/A	N/A	1 milligram
CHLORPHENAMINE (IV/IO/IM) 10 milligrams in 1 ml	2.5 milligrams	NONE	N/A	0.25 ml	2.5 milligrams
DEXAMETHASONE – croup (Oral) 3.8 milligrams per ml (use intravenous preparation orally)	3.8 milligrams	NONE	N/A	1 ml	3.8 milligrams
DIAZEPAM (IV/IO) 10 milligrams in 2 ml	3.5 milligrams	NONE	N/A	0.7 ml	3.5 milligrams
DIAZEPAM (PR) 5 milligrams in 2.5 ml	5 milligrams	NONE	N/A	1 × 5 milligram tube	5 milligrams

Drug Therapy

DRUG	INITIAL DOSE	REPEAT DOSE	DOSE INTERVAL	VOLUME	MAXIMUM DOSE
GLUCAGON (IM) 1 milligram per vial	500 micrograms	NONE	N/A	0.5 vial	500 micrograms
GLUCOSE 10% (IV/IO) 50 grams in 500 ml	2 grams	2 grams	5 minutes	20 ml	6 grams
HYDROCORTISONE (IV/IO/IM) 100 milligrams in 1 ml	50 milligrams	NONE	N/A	0.5 ml	50 milligrams
HYDROCORTISONE (IV/IO/IM) 100 milligrams in 2 ml	50 milligrams	NONE	N/A	1 ml	50 milligrams
IBUPROFEN (Oral) 100 milligrams in 5 ml	100 milligrams	100 milligrams	8 hours	5 ml	300 milligrams
IPRATROPIUM (Neb) 250 micrograms in 1 ml	125 – 250 micrograms	NONE	N/A	0.5 ml – 1 ml	125 – 250 micrograms
IPRATROPIUM (Neb) 500 micrograms in 2 ml	125 – 250 micrograms	NONE	N/A	0.5 ml – 1 ml	125 – 250 micrograms
PATIENT'S OWN MIDAZOLAM* (Buccal) 10 milligrams in 1 ml	5 milligrams	NONE	N/A	0.5 ml	5 milligrams
MORPHINE (IV/IO) 10 milligrams in 10 ml	1 milligram	1 milligram	5 minutes	1 ml	2 milligrams
MORPHINE (Oral) 10 milligrams in 5 ml	2 milligrams	NONE	N/A	1 ml	2 milligrams

Give the dose as prescribed in the child's individualised treatment plan (the dosages described above reflect the recommended dosages for a child of this age).

Drug Therapy

DRUG	INITIAL DOSE	REPEAT DOSE	DOSE INTERVAL	VOLUME	MAXIMUM DOSE
NALOXONE (IV/IO) NB cautions 400 micrograms in 1 ml	120 micrograms	120 micrograms	3 minutes	0.3 ml	1320 micrograms
NALOXONE – INITIAL DOSE (IM) 400 micrograms in 1 ml	120 micrograms	See below	3 minutes	0.3 ml	See below
NALOXONE – REPEAT DOSE (IM) 400 micrograms in 1 ml	–	400 micrograms	–	1 ml	520 micrograms
ONDANSETRON (IV/IO/IM) 2 milligrams in 1 ml	1 milligram	NONE	N/A	0.5 ml	1 milligram
PARACETAMOL (Oral) 120 milligrams in 5 ml – infant suspension	120 milligrams	120 milligrams	4 – 6 hours	5 ml	480 milligrams in 24 hours
PARACETAMOL (IV/IO) 10 milligrams in 1 ml	125 milligrams	125 milligrams	4 – 6 hours	12.5 ml	500 milligrams in 24 hours
SALBUTAMOL (Neb) 2.5 milligrams in 2.5 ml	2.5 milligrams	2.5 milligrams	5 minutes	2.5 ml	No limit
SALBUTAMOL (Neb) 5 milligrams in 2.5 ml	2.5 milligrams	2.5 milligrams	5 minutes	1.25 ml	No limit
TRANEXAMIC ACID (IV) 100 mg/ml	150 mg	NONE	N/A	1.5 ml	150 mg

This page left intentionally blank for your notes

Page for Age

2 YEARS

Vital Signs

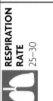 GUIDE WEIGHT	HEART RATE	RESPIRATION RATE	SYSTOLIC BLOOD PRESSURE
12 kg	95–140	25–30	80–100

Airway Size by Type

OROPHARYNGEAL AIRWAY	LARYNGEAL MASK	I-GEL AIRWAY	ENDOTRACHEAL TUBE
0 OR 1	2	1.5 OR 2	Diameter: **5 mm**; Length: **14 cm**

Defibrillation – Cardiac Arrest

MANUAL	AUTOMATED EXTERNAL DEFIBRILLATOR
50 Joules	A standard AED (either with paediatric attenuation pads or else in paediatric mode) can be used. If paediatric pads are not available, standard adult pads can be used (but must not overlap).

Intravascular Fluid

FLUID	INITIAL DOSE	REPEAT DOSE	DOSE INTERVAL	VOLUME	MAXIMUM DOSE
Sodium chloride (5 ml/kg) (IV/IO) 0.9%	60 ml	60 ml	PRN	60 ml	480 ml
Sodium chloride (10 ml/kg) (IV/IO) 0.9%	120 ml	120 ml	PRN	120 ml	480 ml
Sodium chloride (20 ml/kg) (IV/IO) 0.9%	240 ml	240 ml	PRN	240 ml	480 ml

2 YEARS Page for Age

DRUG	INITIAL DOSE	REPEAT DOSE	DOSE INTERVAL	VOLUME	MAXIMUM DOSE
ADRENALINE (IV/IO) 1 milligram in 10 ml (1:10,000)	120 micrograms	120 micrograms	3–5 mins	1.2 ml	No limit
AMIODARONE (IV/IO) 300 milligrams in 10 ml	60 milligrams (after 3rd shock)	60 milligrams	After 5th shock	2 ml	120 milligrams
ATROPINE* (IV/IO) 100 micrograms in 1 ml	240 micrograms	NONE	N/A	2.4 ml	240 micrograms
ATROPINE* (IV/IO) 200 micrograms in 1 ml	240 micrograms	NONE	N/A	1.2 ml	240 micrograms
ATROPINE* (IV/IO) 300 micrograms in 1 ml	240 micrograms	NONE	N/A	0.8 ml	240 micrograms
ATROPINE* (IV/IO) 600 micrograms in 1 ml	240 micrograms	NONE	N/A	0.4 ml	240 micrograms

***BRADYCARDIA** in children is most commonly caused by **HYPOXIA**, requiring immediate **ABC** care, **NOT** drug therapy; therefore **ONLY** administer atropine in cases of bradycardia caused by vagal stimulation (e.g. suction).

Drug Therapy

DRUG	INITIAL DOSE	REPEAT DOSE	DOSE INTERVAL	VOLUME	MAXIMUM DOSE
ADRENALINE (IM) anaphylaxis/asthma 1 milligram in 1 ml (1:1,000)	150 micrograms	150 micrograms	5 minutes	0.15 ml	No limit
BENZYLPENICILLIN (IV/IO) 600 milligrams in 9.6 ml	600 milligrams	NONE	N/A	10 ml	600 milligrams
BENZYLPENICILLIN (IM) 600 milligrams in 1.6 ml	600 milligrams	NONE	N/A	2 ml	600 milligrams
CHLORPHENAMINE (Oral) Various	1 milligram	NONE	N/A	N/A	1 milligram
CHLORPHENAMINE (IV/IO/IM) 10 milligrams in 1 ml	2.5 milligrams	NONE	N/A	0.25 ml	2.5 milligrams
DEXAMETHASONE – croup (Oral) 3.8 milligrams per ml (use intravenous preparation orally)	3.8 milligrams	NONE	N/A	1 ml	3.8 milligrams
DIAZEPAM (IV/IO) 10 milligrams in 2 ml	3.5 milligrams	NONE	N/A	0.7 ml	3.5 milligrams
DIAZEPAM (PR) 5 milligrams in 2.5 ml or 10 milligrams in 2.5 ml	5 or 10 milligrams	NONE	N/A	1 × 5 milligram tube or 1 × 10 milligram tube	5 or 10 milligrams

Drug Therapy

DRUG	INITIAL DOSE	REPEAT DOSE	DOSE INTERVAL	VOLUME	MAXIMUM DOSE
GLUCAGON (IM) 1 milligram per vial	500 micrograms	NONE	N/A	0.5 vial	500 micrograms
GLUCOSE 10% (IV/IO) 50 grams in 500 ml	2.5 grams	2.5 grams	5 minutes	25 ml	7.5 grams
HYDROCORTISONE (IV/IO/IM) 100 milligrams in 1 ml	50 milligrams	NONE	N/A	0.5 ml	50 milligrams
HYDROCORTISONE (IV/IO/IM) 100 milligrams in 2 ml	50 milligrams	NONE	N/A	1 ml	50 milligrams
IBUPROFEN (Oral) 100 milligrams in 5 ml	100 milligrams	100 milligrams	8 hours	5 ml	300 milligrams
IPRATROPIUM (Neb) 250 micrograms in 1 ml	250 micrograms	NONE	N/A	1 ml	250 micrograms
IPRATROPIUM (Neb) 500 micrograms in 2 ml	250 micrograms	NONE	N/A	1 ml	250 micrograms
PATIENT'S OWN **MIDAZOLAM*** (Buccal) 10 milligrams in 1 ml	5 milligrams	NONE	N/A	0.5 ml	5 milligrams
MORPHINE (IV/IO) 10 milligrams in 10 ml	1 milligram	1 milligram	5 minutes	1 ml	2 milligrams
MORPHINE (Oral) 10 milligrams in 5 ml	2 milligrams	NONE	N/A	1 ml	2 milligrams

Give the dose as prescribed in the child's individualised treatment plan (the dosages described above reflect the recommended dosages for a child of this age).

Drug Therapy

2 YEARS Page for Age

DRUG	INITIAL DOSE	REPEAT DOSE	DOSE INTERVAL	VOLUME	MAXIMUM DOSE
NALOXONE (IV/IO) NB cautions 400 micrograms in 1 ml	120 micrograms	120 micrograms	3 minutes	0.3 ml	1320 micrograms
NALOXONE – INITIAL DOSE (IM) 400 micrograms in 1 ml	120 micrograms	See below	3 minutes	0.3 ml	See below
NALOXONE – REPEAT DOSE (IM) 400 micrograms in 1 ml	–	400 micrograms	–	1 ml	520 micrograms
ONDANSETRON (IV/IO/IM) 2 milligrams in 1 ml	1 milligram	NONE	N/A	0.5 ml	1 milligram
PARACETAMOL (Oral) 120 milligrams in 5 ml – infant suspension	180 milligrams	180 milligrams	4 – 6 hours	7.5 ml	720 milligrams in 24 hours
PARACETAMOL (IV/IO) 10 milligrams in 1 ml	125 milligrams	125 milligrams	4 – 6 hours	12.5 ml	500 milligrams in 24 hours
SALBUTAMOL (Neb) 2.5 milligrams in 2.5 ml	2.5 milligrams	2.5 milligrams	5 minutes	2.5 ml	No limit
SALBUTAMOL (Neb) 5 milligrams in 2.5 ml	2.5 milligrams	2.5 milligrams	5 minutes	1.25 ml	No limit
TRANEXAMIC ACID (IV) 100 mg/ml	200 mg	NONE	N/A	2 ml	200 mg

This page left intentionally blank for your notes

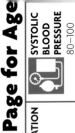

3 YEARS

Page for Age

Vital Signs

GUIDE WEIGHT 14 kg	HEART RATE 95–140	RESPIRATION RATE 25–30	SYSTOLIC BLOOD PRESSURE 80–100

Airway Size by Type

OROPHARYNGEAL AIRWAY	LARYNGEAL MASK	I-GEL AIRWAY	ENDOTRACHEAL TUBE
1	2	2	Diameter: **5 mm**; Length: **14 cm**

Defibrillation – Cardiac Arrest

MANUAL	AUTOMATED EXTERNAL DEFIBRILLATOR
60 Joules	A standard AED (either with paediatric attenuation pads or else in paediatric mode) can be used. If paediatric pads are not available, standard adult pads can be used (but must not overlap).

Intravascular Fluid

FLUID	INITIAL DOSE	REPEAT DOSE	DOSE INTERVAL	VOLUME	MAXIMUM DOSE
Sodium chloride (5 ml/kg) 0.9% (IV/IO)	70 ml	70 ml	PRN	70 ml	560 ml
Sodium chloride (10 ml/kg) 0.9% (IV/IO)	140 ml	140 ml	PRN	140 ml	560 ml
Sodium chloride (20 ml/kg) 0.9% (IV/IO)	280 ml	280 ml	PRN	280 ml	560 ml

3 YEARS   Page for Age

DRUG	INITIAL DOSE	REPEAT DOSE	DOSE INTERVAL	VOLUME	MAXIMUM DOSE
ADRENALINE (IV/IO) 1 milligram in 10 ml (1:10,000)	140 micrograms	140 micrograms	3–5 mins	1.4 ml	No limit
AMIODARONE (IV/IO) 300 milligrams in 10 ml	70 milligrams (after 3rd shock)	70 milligrams	After 5th shock	2.3 ml	140 milligrams
ATROPINE* (IV/IO) 100 micrograms in 1 ml	240 micrograms	NONE	N/A	2.4 ml	240 micrograms
ATROPINE* (IV/IO) 200 micrograms in 1 ml	240 micrograms	NONE	N/A	1.2 ml	240 micrograms
ATROPINE* (IV/IO) 300 micrograms in 1 ml	240 micrograms	NONE	N/A	0.8 ml	240 micrograms
ATROPINE* (IV/IO) 600 micrograms in 1 ml	240 micrograms	NONE	N/A	0.4 ml	240 micrograms

BRADYCARDIA in children is most commonly caused by **HYPOXIA**, requiring immediate **ABC** care. **NOT** drug therapy; therefore **ONLY** administer atropine in cases of bradycardia caused by vagal stimulation (e.g. suction).

Drug Therapy

DRUG	INITIAL DOSE	REPEAT DOSE	DOSE INTERVAL	VOLUME	MAXIMUM DOSE
ADRENALINE (IM) anaphylaxis/asthma 1 milligram in 1 ml (1:1,000)	150 micrograms	150 micrograms	5 minutes	0.15 ml	No limit
BENZYLPENICILLIN (IV/IO) 600 milligrams in 9.6 ml	600 milligrams	NONE	N/A	10 ml	600 milligrams
BENZYLPENICILLIN (IM) 600 milligrams in 1.6 ml	600 milligrams	NONE	N/A	2 ml	600 milligrams
CHLORPHENAMINE (Oral) Various	1 milligram	NONE	N/A	N/A	1 milligram
CHLORPHENAMINE (IV/IO/IM) 10 milligrams in 1 ml	2.5 milligrams	NONE	N/A	0.25 ml	2.5 milligrams
DEXAMETHASONE – croup (Oral) 3.8 milligrams per ml (use intravenous preparation orally)	3.8 milligrams	NONE	N/A	1 ml	3.8 milligrams
DIAZEPAM (IV/IO) 10 milligrams in 2 ml	4.5 milligrams	NONE	N/A	0.9 ml	4.5 milligrams
DIAZEPAM (PR) 5 milligrams in 2.5 ml or 10 milligrams in 2.5 ml	5 or 10 milligrams	NONE	N/A	1 × 5 milligram tube or 1 × 10 milligram tube	5 or 10 milligrams

Drug Therapy

DRUG	INITIAL DOSE	REPEAT DOSE	DOSE INTERVAL	VOLUME	MAXIMUM DOSE
GLUCAGON (IM) 1 milligram per vial	500 micrograms	NONE	N/A	0.5 vial	500 micrograms
GLUCOSE 10% (IV/IO) 50 grams in 500 ml	3 grams	NONE	3 grams	30 ml	9 grams
HYDROCORTISONE (IV/IO/IM) 100 milligrams in 1 ml	50 milligrams	NONE	5 minutes	0.5 ml	50 milligrams
HYDROCORTISONE (IV/IO/IM) 100 milligrams in 2 ml	50 milligrams	NONE	N/A	1 ml	50 milligrams
IBUPROFEN (Oral) 100 milligrams in 5 ml	100 milligrams	100 milligrams	8 hours	5 ml	300 milligrams
IPRATROPIUM (Neb) 250 micrograms in 1 ml	250 micrograms	NONE	N/A	1 ml	250 micrograms
IPRATROPIUM (Neb) 500 micrograms in 2 ml	250 micrograms	NONE	N/A	1 ml	250 micrograms
PATIENT'S OWN MIDAZOLAM* (Buccal) 10 milligrams in 1 ml	5 milligrams	NONE	N/A	0.5 ml	5 milligrams
MORPHINE (IV/IO) 10 milligrams in 10 ml	1.5 milligrams	1.5 milligram	5 minutes	1.5 ml	3 milligrams
MORPHINE (Oral) 10 milligrams in 5 ml	3 milligrams	NONE	N/A	1.5 ml	3 milligrams

Give the dose as prescribed in the child's individualised treatment plan (the dosages described above effect the recommended dosages for a child of this age).

Drug Therapy

DRUG	INITIAL DOSE	REPEAT DOSE	DOSE INTERVAL	VOLUME	MAXIMUM DOSE
NALOXONE (IV/IO) NB cautions 400 micrograms in 1 ml	160 micrograms	160 micrograms	3 minutes	0.4 ml	No limit
NALOXONE **– INITIAL DOSE** (IM) 400 micrograms in 1 ml	160 micrograms	See below	3 minutes	0.4 ml	See below
NALOXONE **– REPEAT DOSE** (IM) 400 micrograms in 1 ml	–	400 micrograms	–	1 ml	560 micrograms
ONDANSETRON (IV/IO/IM) 2 milligrams in 1 ml	1.5 milligrams	NONE	N/A	0.75 ml	1.5 milligrams
PARACETAMOL (Oral) 120 milligrams in 5 ml – infant suspension	180 milligrams	180 milligrams	4 – 6 hours	7.5 ml	720 milligrams in 24 hours
PARACETAMOL (IV/IO) 10 milligrams in 1 ml	250 milligrams	250 milligrams	4 – 6 hours	25 ml	1 gram in 24 hours
SALBUTAMOL (Neb) 2.5 milligrams in 2.5 ml	2.5 milligrams	2.5 milligrams	5 minutes	2.5 ml	No limit
SALBUTAMOL (Neb) 5 milligrams in 2.5 ml	2.5 milligrams	2.5 milligrams	5 minutes	1.25 ml	No limit
TRANEXAMIC ACID (IV) 100 mg/ml	200 mg	NONE	N/A	2 ml	200 mg

This page left intentionally blank for your notes

Page for Age

4 YEARS

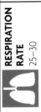

Vital Signs

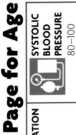 GUIDE WEIGHT 16 kg	HEART RATE 95–140	RESPIRATION RATE 25–30	SYSTOLIC BLOOD PRESSURE 80–100

Airway Size by Type

OROPHARYNGEAL AIRWAY	LARYNGEAL MASK	I-GEL AIRWAY	ENDOTRACHEAL TUBE
1	2	2	Diameter: **5 mm**; Length: **15 cm**

Defibrillation – Cardiac Arrest

MANUAL	AUTOMATED EXTERNAL DEFIBRILLATOR
70 Joules	A standard AED (either with paediatric attenuation pads or else in paediatric mode) can be used. If paediatric pads are not available, standard adult pads can be used (but must not overlap).

Intravascular Fluid

FLUID	INITIAL DOSE	REPEAT DOSE	DOSE INTERVAL	VOLUME	MAXIMUM DOSE
Sodium chloride (5 ml/kg) 0.9% (IV/IO)	80 ml	80 ml	PRN	80 ml	640 ml
Sodium chloride (10 ml/kg) 0.9% (IV/IO)	160 ml	160 ml	PRN	160 ml	640 ml
Sodium chloride (20 ml/kg) 0.9% (IV/IO)	320 ml	320 ml	PRN	320 ml	640 ml

DRUG	INITIAL DOSE	REPEAT DOSE	DOSE INTERVAL	VOLUME	MAXIMUM DOSE
ADRENALINE (IV/IO) 1 milligram in 10 ml (1:10,000)	160 micrograms	160 micrograms	3–5 mins	1.6 ml	No limit
AMIODARONE (IV/IO) 300 milligrams in 10 ml	80 milligrams (after 3rd shock)	80 milligrams	After 5th shock	2.7 ml	160 milligrams
ATROPINE* (IV/IO) 100 micrograms in 1 ml	300 micrograms	NONE	N/A	3 ml	300 micrograms
ATROPINE* (IV/IO) 200 micrograms in 1 ml	300 micrograms	NONE	N/A	1.5 ml	300 micrograms
ATROPINE* (IV/IO) 300 micrograms in 1 ml	300 micrograms	NONE	N/A	1 ml	300 micrograms
ATROPINE* (IV/IO) 600 micrograms in 1 ml	300 micrograms	NONE	N/A	0.5 ml	300 micrograms

*BRADYCARDIA** in children is most commonly caused by **HYPOXIA**, requiring immediate **ABC** care, **NOT** drug therapy; therefore **ONLY** administer atropine in cases of bradycardia caused by vagal stimulation (e.g. suction).

Drug Therapy

4 YEARS Page for Age

DRUG	INITIAL DOSE	REPEAT DOSE	DOSE INTERVAL	VOLUME	MAXIMUM DOSE
ADRENALINE (IM) anaphylaxis/asthma 1 milligram in 1 ml (1:1,000)	150 micrograms	150 micrograms	5 minutes	0.15 ml	No limit
BENZYLPENICILLIN (IV/IO) 600 milligrams in 9.6 ml	600 milligrams	NONE	N/A	10 ml	600 milligrams
BENZYLPENICILLIN (IM) 600 milligrams in 1.6 ml	600 milligrams	NONE	N/A	2 ml	600 milligrams
CHLORPHENAMINE (Oral) Various	1 milligram	NONE	N/A	N/A	1 milligram
CHLORPHENAMINE (IV/IO/IM) 10 milligrams in 1 ml	2.5 milligrams	NONE	N/A	0.25 ml	2.5 milligrams
DEXAMETHASONE – croup (Oral) 3.8 milligrams per ml (use intravenous preparation orally)	3.8 milligrams	NONE	N/A	1 ml	3.8 milligrams
DIAZEPAM (IV/IO) 10 milligrams in 2 ml	5 milligrams	NONE	N/A	1 ml	5 milligrams
DIAZEPAM (PR) 5 milligrams in 2.5 ml or 10 milligrams in 2.5 ml	5 or 10 milligrams	NONE	N/A	1 × 5 milligram tube or 1 × 10 milligram tube	5 or 10 milligrams

Drug Therapy

DRUG	INITIAL DOSE	REPEAT DOSE	DOSE INTERVAL	VOLUME	MAXIMUM DOSE
GLUCAGON (IM) 1 milligram per vial	500 micrograms	NONE	N/A	0.5 vial	500 micrograms
GLUCOSE 10% (IV/IO) 50 grams in 500 ml	3 grams	3 grams	5 minutes	30 ml	9 grams
HYDROCORTISONE (IV/IO/IM) 100 milligrams in 1 ml	50 milligrams	NONE	N/A	0.5 ml	50 milligrams
HYDROCORTISONE (IV/IO/IM) 100 milligrams in 2 ml	50 milligrams	NONE	N/A	1 ml	50 milligrams
IBUPROFEN (Oral) 100 milligrams in 5 ml	150 milligrams	150 milligrams	8 hours	7.5 ml	450 milligrams
IPRATROPIUM (Neb) 250 micrograms in 1 ml	250 micrograms	NONE	N/A	1 ml	250 micrograms
IPRATROPIUM (Neb) 500 micrograms in 2 ml	250 micrograms	NONE	N/A	1 ml	250 micrograms
PATIENT'S OWN MIDAZOLAM* (Buccal) 10 milligrams in 1 ml	5 milligrams	NONE	N/A	0.5 ml	5 milligrams
MORPHINE (IV/IO) 10 milligrams in 10 ml	1.5 milligrams	1.5 milligrams	5 minutes	1.5 ml	3 milligrams
MORPHINE (Oral) 10 milligrams in 5 ml	3 milligrams	NONE	N/A	1.5 ml	3 milligrams

*Give the dose as prescribed in the child's individualised treatment plan (the dosages described above reflect the recommended dosages for a child of this age).

Drug Therapy

4 YEARS — Page for Age

DRUG	INITIAL DOSE	REPEAT DOSE	DOSE INTERVAL	VOLUME	MAXIMUM DOSE
NALOXONE (IV/IO) NB cautions 400 micrograms in 1 ml	160 micrograms	160 micrograms	3 minutes	0.4ml	1760 micrograms
NALOXONE – INITIAL DOSE (IM) 400 micrograms in 1 ml	160 micrograms	See below	3 minutes	0.4 ml	See below
NALOXONE – REPEAT DOSE (IM) 400 micrograms in 1 ml	–	400 micrograms	–	1 ml	560 micrograms
ONDANSETRON (IV/IO/IM) 2 milligrams in 1 ml	1.5 milligrams	NONE	N/A	0.75 ml	1.5 milligrams
PARACETAMOL (Oral) 120 milligrams in 5 ml – infant suspension	240 milligrams	240 milligrams	4 – 6 hours	10 ml	960 milligrams in 24 hours
PARACETAMOL (IV/IO) 10 milligrams in 1 ml	250 milligrams	250 milligrams	4 – 6 hours	25 ml	1 gram in 24 hours
SALBUTAMOL (Neb) 2.5 milligrams in 2.5 ml	2.5 milligrams	2.5 milligrams	5 minutes	2.5 ml	No limit
SALBUTAMOL (Neb) 5 milligrams in 2.5 ml	2.5 milligrams	2.5 milligrams	5 minutes	1.25 ml	No limit
TRANEXAMIC ACID (IV) 100 mg/ml	250 mg	NONE	N/A	2.5 ml	250 mg

This page left intentionally blank for your notes

Page for Age

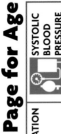

5 YEARS

Vital Signs

GUIDE WEIGHT 19 kg	HEART RATE 80–120	RESPIRATION RATE 20–25	SYSTOLIC BLOOD PRESSURE 90–100

Airway Size by Type

OROPHARYNGEAL AIRWAY	LARYNGEAL MASK	I-GEL AIRWAY	ENDOTRACHEAL TUBE
1	2	2	Diameter: **5.5 mm**; Length: **15 cm**

Defibrillation – Cardiac Arrest

MANUAL	AUTOMATED EXTERNAL DEFIBRILLATOR
80 Joules	A standard AED (either with paediatric attenuation pads or else in paediatric mode) can be used. If paediatric pads are not available, standard adult pads can be used (but must not overlap).

Intravascular Fluid

FLUID	INITIAL DOSE	REPEAT DOSE	DOSE INTERVAL	VOLUME	MAXIMUM DOSE
Sodium chloride (5 ml/kg) 0.9% (IV/IO)	95 ml	95 ml	PRN	95 ml	760 ml
Sodium chloride (10 ml/kg) 0.9% (IV/IO)	190 ml	190 ml	PRN	190 ml	760 ml
Sodium chloride (20 ml/kg) 0.9% (IV/IO)	380 ml	380 ml	PRN	380 ml	760 ml

5 YEARS Page for Age

Cardiac Arrest

DRUG	INITIAL DOSE	REPEAT DOSE	DOSE INTERVAL	VOLUME	MAXIMUM DOSE
ADRENALINE (IV/IO) 1 milligram in 10 ml (1:10,000)	190 micrograms	190 micrograms	3–5 mins	1.9 ml	No limit
AMIODARONE (IV/IO) 300 milligrams in 10 ml	100 milligrams (after 3rd shock)	100 milligrams	After 5th shock	200 milligrams	
ATROPINE* (IV/IO) 100 micrograms in 1 ml	300 micrograms	NONE	N/A	3 ml	300 micrograms
ATROPINE* (IV/IO) 200 micrograms in 1 ml	300 micrograms	NONE	N/A	1.5 ml	300 micrograms
ATROPINE* (IV/IO) 300 micrograms in 1 ml	300 micrograms	NONE	N/A	1 ml	300 micrograms
ATROPINE* (IV/IO) 600 micrograms in 1 ml	300 micrograms	NONE	N/A	0.5 ml	300 micrograms

***BRADYCARDIA** in children is most commonly caused by **HYPOXIA**, requiring immediate **ABC** care, **NOT** drug therapy; therefore **ONLY** administer atropine in cases of bradycardia caused by vagal stimulation (e.g. suction).

5 YEARS Page for Age

Drug Therapy

DRUG	INITIAL DOSE	REPEAT DOSE	DOSE INTERVAL	VOLUME	MAXIMUM DOSE
ADRENALINE (IM) anaphylaxis/asthma 1 milligram in 1 ml (1:1,000)	150 micrograms	150 micrograms	5 minutes	0.15 ml	No limit
BENZYLPENICILLIN (IV/IO) 600 milligrams in 9.6 ml	600 milligrams	NONE	N/A	10 ml	600 milligrams
BENZYLPENICILLIN (IM) 600 milligrams in 1.6 ml	600 milligrams	NONE	N/A	2 ml	600 milligrams
CHLORPHENAMINE (Oral) Various	1 milligram	NONE	N/A	N/A	1 milligram
CHLORPHENAMINE (IV/IO/IM) 10 milligrams in 1 ml	2.5 milligrams	NONE	N/A	0.25 ml	2.5 milligrams
DEXAMETHASONE – croup (Oral) 3.8 milligrams per ml (use intravenous preparation orally)	3.8 milligrams	NONE	N/A	1 ml	3.8 milligrams
DIAZEPAM (IV/IO) 10 milligrams in 2 ml	6 milligrams	NONE	N/A	1.2 ml	6 milligrams
DIAZEPAM (PR) 5 milligrams in 2.5 ml or 10 milligrams in 2.5 ml	5 or 10 milligrams	NONE	N/A	1 × 5 milligram tube or 1 × 10 milligram tube	5 or 10 milligrams

Drug Therapy

DRUG	INITIAL DOSE	REPEAT DOSE	DOSE INTERVAL	VOLUME	MAXIMUM DOSE
GLUCAGON (IM) 1 milligram per vial	500 micrograms	NONE	N/A	0.5 vial	500 micrograms
GLUCOSE 10% (IV/IO) 50 grams in 500 ml	4 grams	4 grams	5 minutes	40 ml	12 grams
HYDROCORTISONE (IV/IO/IM) 100 milligrams in 1 ml	50 milligrams	NONE	N/A	0.5 ml	50 milligrams
HYDROCORTISONE (IV/IO/IM) 100 milligrams in 2 ml	50 milligrams	NONE	N/A	1 ml	50 milligrams
IBUPROFEN (Oral) 100 milligrams in 5 ml	150 milligrams	150 milligrams	8 hours	7.5 ml	450 milligrams
IPRATROPIUM (Neb) 250 micrograms in 1 ml	250 micrograms	NONE	N/A	1 ml	250 micrograms
IPRATROPIUM (Neb) 500 micrograms in 2 ml	250 micrograms	NONE	N/A	1 ml	250 micrograms
PATIENT'S OWN MIDAZOLAM* (Buccal) 10 milligrams in 1 ml	7.5 milligrams	NONE	N/A	0.75 ml	7.5 milligrams
MORPHINE (IV/IO) 10 milligrams in 10 ml	2 milligrams	2 milligrams	5 minutes	2 ml	4 milligrams
MORPHINE (Oral) 10 milligrams in 5 ml	4 milligrams	NONE	N/A	2 ml	4 milligrams

Give the dose as prescribed in the child's individualised treatment plan (the dosages described above reflect the recommended dosages for a child of this age).

Drug Therapy

DRUG	INITIAL DOSE	REPEAT DOSE	DOSE INTERVAL	VOLUME	MAXIMUM DOSE
NALOXONE (IV/IO) NB cautions 400 micrograms in 1 ml	200 micrograms	200 micrograms	3 minutes	0.5 ml	2200 micrograms
NALOXONE – INITIAL DOSE (IM) 400 micrograms in 1 ml	200 micrograms	See below	3 minutes	0.5 ml	See below
NALOXONE – REPEAT DOSE (IM) 400 micrograms in 1 ml	–	400 micrograms	–	1 ml	600 micrograms
ONDANSETRON (IV/IO/IM) 2 milligrams in 1 ml	2 milligrams	NONE	N/A	1 ml	2 milligrams
PARACETAMOL (Oral) 120 milligrams in 5 ml – infant suspension	240 milligrams	240 milligrams	4 – 6 hours	10 ml	960 milligrams in 24 hours
PARACETAMOL (IV/IO) 10 milligrams in 1 ml	250 milligrams	250 milligrams	4 – 6 hours	25 ml	1 gram in 24 hours
SALBUTAMOL (Neb) 2.5 milligrams in 2.5 ml	2.5 milligrams	2.5 milligrams	5 minutes	2.5 ml	No limit
SALBUTAMOL (Neb) 5 milligrams in 2.5 ml	2.5 milligrams	2.5 milligrams	5 minutes	1.25 ml	No limit
TRANEXAMIC ACID (IV) 100 mg/ml	300 mg	NONE	N/A	3 ml	300 mg

This page left intentionally blank for your notes

6 YEARS

Page for Age

Vital Signs

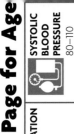

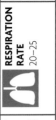 GUIDE WEIGHT 21 kg	HEART RATE 80–120	RESPIRATION RATE 20–25	SYSTOLIC BLOOD PRESSURE 80–110

Airway Size by Type

OROPHARYNGEAL AIRWAY	LARYNGEAL MASK	I-GEL AIRWAY	ENDOTRACHEAL TUBE
1	2.5	2	Diameter: **6 mm**; Length: **16 cm**

Defibrillation – Cardiac Arrest

MANUAL	AUTOMATED EXTERNAL DEFIBRILLATOR
80 Joules	A standard AED (either with paediatric attenuation pads or else in paediatric mode) can be used. If paediatric pads are not available, standard adult pads can be used (but must not overlap).

Intravascular Fluid

FLUID	INITIAL DOSE	REPEAT DOSE	DOSE INTERVAL	VOLUME	MAXIMUM DOSE
Sodium chloride (5 ml/kg) (IV/IO) 0.9%	105 ml	105 ml	PRN	105 ml	840 ml
Sodium chloride (10 ml/kg) (IV/IO) 0.9%	210 ml	210 ml	PRN	210 ml	840 ml
Sodium chloride (20 ml/kg) (IV/IO) 0.9%	420 ml	420 ml	PRN	420 ml	840 ml

6 YEARS — Page for Age

DRUG	INITIAL DOSE	REPEAT DOSE	DOSE INTERVAL	VOLUME	MAXIMUM DOSE
ADRENALINE (IV/IO) 1 milligram in 10 ml (1:10,000)	210 micrograms	210 micrograms	3–5 mins	2.1 ml	No limit
AMIODARONE (IV/IO) 300 milligrams in 10 ml	100 milligrams (after 3rd shock)	100 milligrams	After 5th shock	3.3 ml	200 milligrams
ATROPINE* (IV/IO) 100 micrograms in 1 ml	400 micrograms	NONE	N/A	4 ml	400 micrograms
ATROPINE* (IV/IO) 200 micrograms in 1 ml	400 micrograms	NONE	N/A	2 ml	400 micrograms
ATROPINE* (IV/IO) 300 micrograms in 1 ml	400 micrograms	NONE	N/A	1.3 ml	400 micrograms
ATROPINE* (IV/IO) 600 micrograms in 1 ml	400 micrograms	NONE	N/A	0.7 ml	400 micrograms

*BRADYCARDIA in children is most commonly caused by **HYPOXIA**, requiring immediate **ABC** care, **NOT** drug therapy; therefore **ONLY** administer atropine in cases of bradycardia caused by vagal stimulation (e.g. suction).

Drug Therapy

DRUG	INITIAL DOSE	REPEAT DOSE	DOSE INTERVAL	VOLUME	MAXIMUM DOSE
ADRENALINE (IM) anaphylaxis/asthma 1 milligram in 1 ml (1:1.000)	300 micrograms	300 micrograms	5 minutes	0.3 ml	No limit
BENZYLPENICILLIN (IV/IO) 600 milligrams in 9.6 ml	600 milligrams	NONE	N/A	10 ml	600 milligrams
BENZYLPENICILLIN (IM) 600 milligrams in 1.6 ml	600 milligrams	NONE	N/A	2 ml	600 milligrams
CHLORPHENAMINE (Oral) Various	2 milligrams	NONE	N/A	N/A	2 milligrams
CHLORPHENAMINE (IV/IO/IM) 10 milligrams in 1 ml	5–10 milligrams	NONE	N/A	0.5 – 1 ml	5 – 10 milligrams
DEXAMETHASONE – croup (Oral) 3.8 milligrams per ml (use intravenous preparation orally)	3.8 milligrams	NONE	N/A	1 ml	3.8 milligrams
DIAZEPAM (IV/IO) 10 milligrams in 2 ml	6.5 milligrams	NONE	N/A	1.3 ml	6.5 milligrams
DIAZEPAM (PR) 5 milligrams in 2.5 ml or 10 milligrams in 2.5 ml	5 or 10 milligrams	NONE	N/A	1 × 5 milligram tube or 1 × 10 milligram tube	5 or 10 milligrams

Drug Therapy

DRUG	INITIAL DOSE	REPEAT DOSE	DOSE INTERVAL	VOLUME	MAXIMUM DOSE
GLUCAGON (IM) 1 milligram per vial	500 micrograms	NONE	N/A	0.5 vial	500 micrograms
GLUCOSE 10% (IV/IO) 50 grams in 500 ml	4 grams	4 grams	5 minutes	40 ml	12 grams
HYDROCORTISONE (IV/IO/IM) 100 milligrams in 1 ml	100 milligrams	NONE	N/A	1 ml	100 milligrams
HYDROCORTISONE (IV/IO/IM) 100 milligrams in 2 ml	100 milligrams	NONE	N/A	2 ml	100 milligrams
IBUPROFEN (Oral) 100 milligrams in 5 ml	150 milligrams	150 milligrams	8 hours	7.5 ml	450 milligrams
IPRATROPIUM (Neb) 250 micrograms in 1 ml	250 micrograms	NONE	N/A	1 ml	250 micrograms
IPRATROPIUM (Neb) 500 micrograms in 2 ml	250 micrograms	NONE	N/A	1 ml	250 micrograms
MIDAZOLAM* (Buccal) 10 milligrams in 1 ml	7.5 milligrams	NONE	N/A	0.75 ml	7.5 milligrams
MORPHINE (IV/IO) 10 milligrams in 10 ml	2 milligrams	2 milligrams	5 minutes	2 ml	4 milligrams
MORPHINE (Oral) 10 milligrams in 5 ml	4 milligrams	NONE	N/A	2 ml	4 milligrams

*Give the dose as prescribed in the child's individualised treatment plan (the dosages described above reflect the recommended dosages for a child of this age).

PATIENT'S OWN

DRUG	INITIAL DOSE	REPEAT DOSE	DOSE INTERVAL	VOLUME	MAXIMUM DOSE
NALOXONE (IV/IO) NB cautions 400 micrograms in 1 ml	200 micrograms	200 micrograms	3 minutes	0.5 ml	2200 micrograms
NALOXONE – INITIAL DOSE (IM) 400 micrograms in 1 ml	200 micrograms	See below	3 minutes	0.5 ml	See below
NALOXONE – REPEAT DOSE (IM) 400 micrograms in 1 ml	–	400 micrograms	–	1 ml	600 micrograms
ONDANSETRON (IV/IO/IM) 2 milligrams in 1 ml	2 milligrams	NONE	N/A	1 ml	2 milligrams
PARACETAMOL (Oral) 250 milligrams in 5 ml – six plus suspension	250 milligrams	250 milligrams	4 – 6 hours	5 ml	1 gram in 24 hours
PARACETAMOL (IV/IO) 10 milligrams in 1 ml	300 milligrams	300 milligrams	4 – 6 hours	30 ml	1.2 grams in 24 hours
SALBUTAMOL (Neb) 2.5 milligrams in 2.5 ml	5 milligrams	5 milligrams	5 minutes	5 ml	No limit
SALBUTAMOL (Neb) 5 milligrams in 2.5 ml	5 milligrams	5 milligrams	5 minutes	2.5 ml	No limit
TRANEXAMIC ACID (IV) 100 mg/ml	300 mg	NONE	N/A	3 ml	300 mg

This page left intentionally blank for your notes

Page for Age

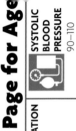

7 YEARS

Vital Signs

GUIDE WEIGHT 23 kg	HEART RATE 80–120	RESPIRATION RATE 20–25	SYSTOLIC BLOOD PRESSURE 90–110

Airway Size by Type

OROPHARYNGEAL AIRWAY	LARYNGEAL MASK	I-GEL AIRWAY	ENDOTRACHEAL TUBE
1 OR 2	2.5	2	Diameter: **6 mm**; Length: **16 cm**

Defibrillation – Cardiac Arrest

MANUAL	AUTOMATED EXTERNAL DEFIBRILLATOR
100 Joules	A standard AED (either with paediatric attenuation pads or else in paediatric mode) can be used. If paediatric pads are not available, standard adult pads can be used (but must not overlap).

Intravascular Fluid

FLUID	INITIAL DOSE	REPEAT DOSE	DOSE INTERVAL	VOLUME	MAXIMUM DOSE
Sodium chloride (5 ml/kg) (IV/IO) 0.9%	115 ml	115 ml	PRN	115 ml	920 ml
Sodium chloride (10 ml/kg) (IV/IO) 0.9%	230 ml	230 ml	PRN	230 ml	920 ml
Sodium chloride (20 ml/kg) (IV/IO) 0.9%	460 ml	460 ml	PRN	460 ml	920 ml

7 YEARS   Page for Age

DRUG	INITIAL DOSE	REPEAT DOSE	DOSE INTERVAL	VOLUME	MAXIMUM DOSE
ADRENALINE (IV/IO) 1 milligram in 10 ml (1:10,000)	230 micrograms	230 micrograms	3–5 mins	2.3 ml	No limit
AMIODARONE (IV/IO) 300 milligrams in 10 ml	120 milligrams (after 3rd shock)	120 milligrams	After 5th shock		240 milligrams
ATROPINE* (IV/IO) 300 micrograms in 1 ml	400 micrograms	NONE	N/A	4 ml	400 micrograms
ATROPINE* (IV/IO) 200 micrograms in 1 ml	400 micrograms	NONE	N/A	2 ml	400 micrograms
ATROPINE* (IV/IO) 300 micrograms in 1 ml	400 micrograms	NONE	N/A	1.3 ml	400 micrograms
ATROPINE* (IV/IO) 600 micrograms in 1 ml	400 micrograms	NONE	N/A	0.7 ml	400 micrograms

BRADYCARDIA in children is most commonly caused by **HYPOXIA**, requiring immediate **ABC** care. **NOT** drug therapy; therefore **ONLY** administer atropine in cases of bradycardia caused by vagal stimulation (e.g. ...uction).

Drug Therapy

DRUG	INITIAL DOSE	REPEAT DOSE	DOSE INTERVAL	VOLUME	MAXIMUM DOSE
ADRENALINE (IM) anaphylaxis/asthma 1 milligram in 1 ml (1:1,000)	300 micrograms	300 micrograms	5 minutes	0.3 ml	No limit
BENZYLPENICILLIN (IV/IO) 600 milligrams in 9.6 ml	600 milligrams	NONE	N/A	10 ml	600 milligrams
BENZYLPENICILLIN (IM) 600 milligrams in 1.6 ml	600 milligrams	NONE	N/A	2 ml	600 milligrams
CHLORPHENAMINE (Oral) Various	2 milligrams	NONE	N/A	N/A	2 milligrams
CHLORPHENAMINE (IV/IO/IM) 10 milligrams in 1 ml	5–10 milligrams	NONE	N/A	0.5 – 1 ml	5 – 10 milligrams
DEXAMETHASONE – croup (Oral)	N/A	NONE	N/A	N/A	N/A
DIAZEPAM (IV/IO) 10 milligrams in 2 ml	7 milligrams	NONE	N/A	1.4 ml	7 milligrams
DIAZEPAM (PR) 5 milligrams in 2.5 ml or 10 milligrams in 2.5 ml	5 or 10 milligrams	NONE	N/A	1 × 5 milligram tube or 1 × 10 milligram tube	5 or 10 milligrams
GLUCAGON (IM) 1 milligram per vial	500 micrograms	NONE	N/A	0.5 vial	500 micrograms

DRUG	INITIAL DOSE	REPEAT DOSE	DOSE INTERVAL	VOLUME	MAXIMUM DOSE
GLUCOSE 10% (IV/IO) 50 grams in 500 ml	5 grams	5 grams	5 minutes	50 ml	15 grams
HYDROCORTISONE (IV/IO/IM) 100 milligrams in 1 ml	100 milligrams	NONE	N/A	1 ml	100 milligrams
HYDROCORTISONE (IV/IO/IM) 100 milligrams in 2 ml	100 milligrams	NONE	N/A	2 ml	100 milligrams
IBUPROFEN (Oral) 100 milligrams in 5 ml	200 milligrams	200 milligrams	8 hours	10 ml	600 milligrams
IPRATROPIUM (Neb) 250 micrograms in 1 ml	250 micrograms	NONE	N/A	1 ml	250 micrograms
IPRATROPIUM (Neb) 500 micrograms in 2 ml	250 micrograms	NONE	N/A	1 ml	250 micrograms
PATIENT'S OWN MIDAZOLAM* (Buccal) 10 milligrams in 1 ml	7.5 milligrams	NONE	N/A	0.75 ml	7.5 milligrams
MORPHINE (IV/IO) 10 milligrams in 10 ml	2.5 milligrams	2.5 milligrams	5 minutes	2.5 ml	5 milligrams
MORPHINE (Oral) 10 milligrams in 5 ml	5 milligrams	NONE	N/A	2.5 ml	5 milligrams

Give the dose as prescribed in the child's individualised treatment plan (the dosages described above reflect the recommended dosages for a child of this age).

Drug Therapy

DRUG	INITIAL DOSE	REPEAT DOSE	DOSE INTERVAL	VOLUME	MAXIMUM DOSE
NALOXONE (IV/IO) NB cautions 400 micrograms in 1 ml	240 micrograms	240 micrograms	3 minutes	0.6 ml	2640 micrograms
NALOXONE **– INITIAL DOSE** (IM) 400 micrograms in 1 ml	240 micrograms	See below	3 minutes	0.6 ml	See below
NALOXONE **– REPEAT DOSE** (IM) 400 micrograms in 1 ml	–	400 micrograms	–	1 ml	640 micrograms
ONDANSETRON (IV/IO/IM) 2 milligrams in 1 ml	2.5 milligrams	NONE	N/A	1.3 ml	2.5 milligrams
PARACETAMOL (Oral) 250 milligrams in 5 ml – six plus suspension	250 milligrams	250 milligrams	4 – 6 hours	5 ml	1 gram in 24 hours
PARACETAMOL (IV/IO) 10 milligrams in 1 ml	300 milligrams	300 milligrams	4 – 6 hours	30 ml	1.2 grams in 24 hours
SALBUTAMOL (Neb) 2.5 milligrams in 2.5 ml	5 milligrams	5 milligrams	5 minutes	5 ml	No limit
SALBUTAMOL (Neb) 5 milligrams in 2.5 ml	5 milligrams	5 milligrams	5 minutes	2.5 ml	No limit
TRANEXAMIC ACID (IV) 100 mg/ml	350 mg	NONE	N/A	3.5 ml	350 mg

This page left intentionally blank for your notes

Page for Age

8 YEARS

Vital Signs

GUIDE WEIGHT 26 kg	HEART RATE 80–120	RESPIRATION RATE 20–25	SYSTOLIC BLOOD PRESSURE 90–110

Airway Size by Type

OROPHARYNGEAL AIRWAY	LARYNGEAL MASK	I-GEL AIRWAY	ENDOTRACHEAL TUBE
1 OR 2	2.5	2.5	Diameter: **6.5 mm**; Length: **17 cm**

Defibrillation – Cardiac Arrest

MANUAL	AUTOMATED EXTERNAL DEFIBRILLATOR
100 Joules	A standard AED (either with paediatric attenuation pads or else in paediatric mode) can be used. If paediatric pads are not available, standard adult pads can be used (but must not overlap).

Intravascular Fluid

FLUID	INITIAL DOSE	REPEAT DOSE	DOSE INTERVAL	VOLUME	MAXIMUM DOSE
Sodium chloride (5 ml/kg) (IV/IO) 0.9%	130 ml	130 ml	PRN	130 ml	1000 ml
Sodium chloride (10 ml/kg) (IV/IO) 0.9%	250 ml	250 ml	PRN	250 ml	1000 ml
Sodium chloride (20 ml/kg) (IV/IO) 0.9%	500 ml	500 ml	PRN	500 ml	1000 ml

8 YEARS Page for Age

DRUG	INITIAL DOSE	REPEAT DOSE	DOSE INTERVAL	VOLUME	MAXIMUM DOSE
ADRENALINE (IV/IO) 1 milligram in 10 ml (1:10,000)	260 micrograms	230 micrograms	3–5 mins	2.6 ml	No limit
AMIODARONE (IV/IO) 300 milligrams in 10 ml	130 milligrams (after 3rd shock)	130 milligrams	After 5th shock	4.3 ml	260 milligrams
ATROPINE* (IV/IO) 100 micrograms in 1 ml	500 micrograms	NONE	N/A	5 ml	500 micrograms
ATROPINE* (IV/IO) 200 micrograms in 1 ml	500 micrograms	NONE	N/A	2.5 ml	500 micrograms
ATROPINE* (IV/IO) 300 micrograms in 1 ml	500 micrograms	NONE	N/A	1.7 ml	500 micrograms
ATROPINE* (IV/IO) 600 micrograms in 1 ml	500 micrograms	NONE	N/A	0.8 ml	500 micrograms

*BRADYCARDIA in children is most commonly caused by **HYPOXIA**, requiring immediate **ABC** care, **NOT** drug therapy; therefore **ONLY** administer atropine in cases of bradycardia caused by vagal stimulation (e.g. suction).

Drug Therapy

8 YEARS Page for Age

DRUG	INITIAL DOSE	REPEAT DOSE	DOSE INTERVAL	VOLUME	MAXIMUM DOSE
ADRENALINE (IM) anaphylaxis/asthma 1 milligram in 1 ml (1:1,000)	300 micrograms	300 micrograms	5 minutes	0.3 ml	No limit
BENZYLPENICILLIN (IV/IO) 600 milligrams in 9.6 ml	600 milligrams	NONE	N/A	10 ml	600 milligrams
BENZYLPENICILLIN (IM) 600 milligrams in 1.6 ml	600 milligrams	NONE	N/A	2 ml	600 milligrams
CHLORPHENAMINE (Oral) Various	2 milligrams	NONE	N/A	N/A	2 milligrams
CHLORPHENAMINE (IV/IO/IM) 10 milligrams in 1 ml	5 – 10 milligrams	NONE	N/A	0.5 – 1 ml	5 – 10 milligrams
DEXAMETHASONE – croup (Oral)	N/A	N/A	N/A	N/A	N/A
DIAZEPAM (IV/IO) 10 milligrams in 2 ml	8 milligrams	NONE	N/A	1.6 ml	8 milligrams
DIAZEPAM (PR) 5 milligrams in 2.5 ml or 10 milligrams in 2.5 ml	5 or 10 milligrams	NONE	N/A	1 × 5 milligram tube or 1 × 10 milligram tube	5 or 10 milligrams
GLUCAGON (IM) 1 milligram per vial	1 milligram	NONE	N/A	1 vial	1 milligram

DRUG	INITIAL DOSE	REPEAT DOSE	DOSE INTERVAL	VOLUME	MAXIMUM DOSE
GLUCOSE 10% (IV/IO) 50 grams in 500 ml	5 grams	5 grams	5 minutes	50 ml	15 grams
HYDROCORTISONE (IV/IO/IM) 100 milligrams in 1 ml	100 milligrams	NONE	N/A	1 ml	100 milligrams
HYDROCORTISONE (IV/IO/IM) 100 milligrams in 2 ml	100 milligrams	NONE	N/A	2 ml	100 milligrams
IBUPROFEN (Oral) 100 milligrams in 5 ml	200 milligrams	200 milligrams	8 hours	10 ml	600 milligrams
IPRATROPIUM (Neb) 250 micrograms in 1 ml	250 micrograms	NONE	N/A	1 ml	250 micrograms
IPRATROPIUM (Neb) 500 micrograms in 2 ml	250 micrograms	NONE	N/A	1 ml	250 micrograms
PATIENT'S OWN MIDAZOLAM* (Buccal) 10 milligrams in 1 m	7.5 milligrams	NONE	N/A	0.75 ml	7.5 milligrams
MORPHINE (IV/IO) 10 milligrams in 10 ml	2.5 milligrams	2.5 milligrams	5 minutes	2.5 ml	5 milligrams
MORPHINE (Oral) 10 milligrams in 5 ml	5 milligrams	NONE	N/A	2.5 ml	5 milligrams

*Give the dose as prescribed in the child's individualised treatment plan (the dosages described above reflect the recommended dosages for a child of this age).

DRUG	INITIAL DOSE	REPEAT DOSE	DOSE INTERVAL	VOLUME	MAXIMUM DOSE
NALOXONE (IV/IO) NB cautions 400 micrograms in 1 ml	280 micrograms	280 micrograms	3 minutes	0.7ml	3080 micrograms
NALOXONE – INITIAL DOSE (IM) 400 micrograms in 1 ml	280 micrograms	See below	3 minutes	0.7 ml	See below
NALOXONE – REPEAT DOSE (IM) 400 micrograms in 1 ml	–	400 micrograms	–	1 ml	680 micrograms
ONDANSETRON (IV/IO/IM) 2 milligrams in 1 ml	2.5 milligrams	NONE	N/A	1.3 ml	2.5 milligrams
PARACETAMOL (Oral) 250 milligrams in 5 ml – six plus suspension	375 milligrams	375 milligrams	4 – 6 hours	7.5 ml	1.5 grams in 24 hours
PARACETAMOL (IV/IO) 10 milligrams in 1 ml	300 milligrams	300 milligrams	4 – 6 hours	30 ml	1.2 grams in 24 hours
SALBUTAMOL (Neb) 2.5 milligrams in 2.5 ml	5 milligrams	5 milligrams	5 minutes	5 ml	No limit
SALBUTAMOL (Neb) 5 milligrams in 2.5 ml	5 milligrams	5 milligrams	5 minutes	2.5 ml	No limit
TRANEXAMIC ACID (IV) 100 mg/ml	400 mg	NONE	N/A	4 ml	400 mg

This page left intentionally blank for your notes

9 YEARS

Vital Signs

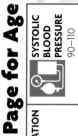

GUIDE WEIGHT 29 kg	HEART RATE 80–120	RESPIRATION RATE 20–25	SYSTOLIC BLOOD PRESSURE 90–110

Airway Size by Type

OROPHARYNGEAL AIRWAY	LARYNGEAL MASK	I-GEL AIRWAY	ENDOTRACHEAL TUBE
1 OR 2	2.5	2.5	Diameter: **6.5 mm**; Length: **17 cm**

Defibrillation – Cardiac Arrest

MANUAL	AUTOMATED EXTERNAL DEFIBRILLATOR
120 Joules	A standard AED can be used (without the need for attenuation pads).

Intravascular Fluid

FLUID	INITIAL DOSE	REPEAT DOSE	DOSE INTERVAL	VOLUME	MAXIMUM DOSE
Sodium chloride (5 ml/kg) (IV/IO) 0.9%	145 ml	145 ml	PRN	145 ml	1000 ml
Sodium chloride (10 ml/kg) (IV/IO) 0.9%	290 ml	290 ml	PRN	290 ml	1000 ml
Sodium chloride (20 ml/kg) (IV/IO) 0.9%	500 ml	500 ml	PRN	500 ml	1000 ml

DRUG	INITIAL DOSE	REPEAT DOSE	DOSE INTERVAL	VOLUME	MAXIMUM DOSE
ADRENALINE (IV/IO) 1 milligram in 10 ml (1:10,000)	300 micrograms	300 micrograms	3–5 mins	3 ml	No limit
AMIODARONE (IV/IO) 300 milligrams in 10 ml	150 milligrams (after 3rd shock)	150 milligrams	After 5th shock	5 ml	300 milligrams
ATROPINE* (IV/IO) 100 micrograms in 1 ml	500 micrograms	NONE	N/A	5 ml	300 micrograms
ATROPINE* (IV/IO) 200 micrograms in 1 ml	500 micrograms	NONE	N/A	2.5 ml	500 micrograms
ATROPINE* (IV/IO) 300 micrograms in 1 ml	500 micrograms	NONE	N/A	1.7 ml	500 micrograms
ATROPINE* (IV/IO) 600 micrograms in 1 ml	500 micrograms	NONE	N/A	0.8 ml	500 micrograms

***BRADYCARDIA** in children is most commonly caused by **HYPOXIA**, requiring immediate **ABC** care, **NOT** drug therapy; therefore **ONLY** administer atropine in cases of bradycardia caused by vagal stimulation (e.g. suction).

Drug Therapy

DRUG	INITIAL DOSE	REPEAT DOSE	DOSE INTERVAL	VOLUME	MAXIMUM DOSE
ADRENALINE (IM) anaphylaxis/asthma 1 milligram in 1 ml (1:1,000)	300 micrograms	300 micrograms	5 minutes	0.3 ml	No limit
BENZYLPENICILLIN (IV/IO) 600 milligrams in 9.6 ml	600 milligrams	NONE	N/A	10 ml	600 milligrams
BENZYLPENICILLIN (IM) 600 milligrams in 1.6 ml	600 milligrams	NONE	N/A	2 ml	600 milligrams
CHLORPHENAMINE (Oral) Various	2 milligrams	NONE	N/A	N/A	2 milligrams
CHLORPHENAMINE (IV/IO/IM) 10 milligrams in 1 ml	5–10 milligrams	NONE	N/A	0.5 – 1 ml	5 – 10 milligrams
DEXAMETHASONE – croup (Oral)	N/A	N/A	N/A	N/A	N/A
DIAZEPAM (IV/IO) 10 milligrams in 2 ml	9 milligrams	NONE	N/A	1.8 ml	9 milligrams
DIAZEPAM (PR) 5 milligrams in 2.5 ml or 10 milligrams in 2.5 ml	5 or 10 milligrams	NONE	N/A	1 × 5 milligram tube or 1 × 10 milligram tube	5 or 10 milligrams
GLUCAGON (IM) 1 milligram per vial	1 milligram	NONE	N/A	1 vial	1 milligram

Drug Therapy

9 YEARS Page for Age

DRUG	INITIAL DOSE	REPEAT DOSE	DOSE INTERVAL	VOLUME	MAXIMUM DOSE
GLUCOSE 10% (IV/IO) 50 grams in 500 ml	6 grams	6 grams	5 minutes	60 ml	18 grams
HYDROCORTISONE (IV/IO/IM) 100 milligrams in 1 ml	100 milligrams	NONE	N/A	1 ml	100 milligrams
HYDROCORTISONE (IV/IO/IM) 100 milligrams in 2 ml	100 milligrams	NONE	N/A	2 ml	100 milligrams
IBUPROFEN (Oral) 100 milligrams in 5 ml	200 milligrams	200 milligrams	8 hours	10 ml	600 milligrams
IPRATROPIUM (Neb) 250 micrograms in 1 ml	250 micrograms	NONE	N/A	1 ml	250 micrograms
IPRATROPIUM (Neb) 500 micrograms in 2 ml	250 micrograms	NONE	N/A	1 ml	250 micrograms
PATIENT'S OWN MIDAZOLAM* (Buccal) 10 milligrams in 1 ml	7.5 milligrams	NONE	N/A	0.75 ml	7.5 milligrams
MORPHINE (IV/IO) 10 milligrams in 10 ml	3 milligrams	3 milligrams	5 minutes	3 ml	6 milligrams
MORPHINE (Oral) 10 milligrams in 5 ml	6 milligrams	NONE	N/A	3 ml	6 milligrams

*Give the dose as prescribed in the child's individualised treatment plan (the dosages described above reflect the recommended dosages for a child of this age).

Drug Therapy

DRUG	INITIAL DOSE	REPEAT DOSE	DOSE INTERVAL	VOLUME	MAXIMUM DOSE
NALOXONE (IV/IO) NB cautions 400 micrograms in 1 ml	280 micrograms	280 micrograms	3 minutes	0.7ml	3080 micrograms
NALOXONE – INITIAL DOSE (IM) 400 micrograms in 1 ml	280 micrograms	See below	3 minutes	0.7 ml	See below
NALOXONE – REPEAT DOSE (IM) 400 micrograms in 1 ml	–	400 micrograms	–	1 ml	680 micrograms
ONDANSETRON (IV/IO/IM) 2 milligrams in 1 ml	3 milligrams	NONE	N/A	1.5 ml	3 milligrams
PARACETAMOL (Oral) 250 milligrams in 5 ml – six plus suspension	375 milligrams	375 milligrams	4 – 6 hours	7.5 ml	1.5 grams in 24 hours
PARACETAMOL (IV/IO) 10 milligrams in 1 ml	500 milligrams	500 milligrams	4 – 6 hours	50 ml	2 grams in 24 hours
SALBUTAMOL (Neb) 2.5 milligrams in 2.5 ml	5 milligrams	5 milligrams	5 minutes	5 ml	No limit
SALBUTAMOL (Neb) 5 milligrams in 2.5 ml	5 milligrams	5 milligrams	5 minutes	2.5 ml	No limit
TRANEXAMIC ACID (IV) 100 mg/ml	450 mg	NONE	N/A	4.5 ml	450 mg

This page left intentionally blank for your notes

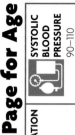

Page for Age

10 YEARS

Vital Signs

GUIDE WEIGHT	HEART RATE	RESPIRATION RATE	SYSTOLIC BLOOD PRESSURE
32 kg	80–120	20–25	90–110

Airway Size by Type

OROPHARYNGEAL AIRWAY	LARYNGEAL MASK	I-GEL AIRWAY	ENDOTRACHEAL TUBE
2 OR 3	3	2.5 OR 3	Diameter: **7 mm**; Length: **18 cm**

Defibrillation – Cardiac Arrest

MANUAL	AUTOMATED EXTERNAL DEFIBRILLATOR
130 Joules	A standard AED can be used (without the need for attenuation pads).

Intravascular Fluid

FLUID	INITIAL DOSE	REPEAT DOSE	DOSE INTERVAL	VOLUME	MAXIMUM DOSE
Sodium chloride (5 ml/kg) (IV/IO) 0.9%	160 ml	160 ml	PRN	160 ml	1000 ml
Sodium chloride (10 ml/kg) (IV/IO) 0.9%	320 ml	320 ml	PRN	320 ml	1000 ml
Sodium chloride (20 ml/kg) (IV/IO) 0.9%	500 ml	500 ml	PRN	500 ml	1000 ml

DRUG	INITIAL DOSE	REPEAT DOSE	DOSE INTERVAL	VOLUME	MAXIMUM DOSE
ADRENALINE (IV/IO) 1 milligram in 10 ml (1:10,000)	320 micrograms	320 micrograms	3–5 mins	3.2 ml	No limit
AMIODARONE (IV/IO) 300 milligrams in 10 ml	160 milligrams (after 3rd shock)	160 milligrams	After 5th shock	5.3 ml	320 milligrams
ATROPINE* (IV/IO) 100 micrograms in 1 ml	500 micrograms	NONE	N/A	5 ml	500 micrograms
ATROPINE* (IV/IO) 200 micrograms in 1 ml	500 micrograms	NONE	N/A	2.5 ml	500 micrograms
ATROPINE* (IV/IO) 300 micrograms in 1 ml	500 micrograms	NONE	N/A	1.7 ml	500 micrograms
ATROPINE* (IV/IO) 600 micrograms in 1 ml	500 micrograms	NONE	N/A	0.8 ml	500 micrograms

*****BRADYCARDIA** in children is most commonly caused by **HYPOXIA**, requiring immediate **ABC** care. **NOT** drug therapy; therefore **ONLY** administer atropine in cases of bradycardia caused by vagal stimulation (e.g. suction).

Drug Therapy

DRUG	INITIAL DOSE	REPEAT DOSE	DOSE INTERVAL	VOLUME DOSE	MAXIMUM
ADRENALINE (IM) anaphylaxis/asthma 1 milligram in 1 ml (1:1,000)	300 micrograms	300 micrograms	5 minutes	0.3 ml	No limit
BENZYLPENICILLIN (IV/IO) 600 milligrams in 9.6 ml	1.2 grams	NONE	N/A	20 ml	1.2 grams
BENZYLPENICILLIN (IM) 600 milligrams in 1.6 ml	1.2 grams	NONE	N/A	4 ml	1.2 grams
CHLORPHENAMINE (Oral) Various	2 milligrams	NONE	N/A	N/A	2 milligrams
CHLORPHENAMINE (IV/IO/IM) 10 milligrams in 1 ml	5–10 milligrams	NONE	N/A	0.5 – 1 ml milligrams	5 – 10
DEXAMETHASONE – croup (Oral)	N/A	N/A	N/A	N/A	N/A
DIAZEPAM (IV/IO) 10 milligrams in 2 ml	10 milligrams	NONE	N/A	2 ml	10 milligrams
DIAZEPAM (PR) 5 milligrams in 2.5 ml or 10 milligrams in 2.5 ml	5 or 10 milligrams	NONE	N/A	1 × 5 milligram tube or 1 × 10 milligram tube	5 or 10 milligrams
GLUCAGON (IM) 1 milligram per vial	1 milligram	NONE	N/A	1 vial	1 milligram

10 YEARS Page for Age

DRUG	INITIAL DOSE	REPEAT DOSE	DOSE INTERVAL	VOLUME	MAXIMUM DOSE
GLUCOSE 10% (IV/IO) 50 grams in 500 ml	6.5 grams	6.5 grams	5 minutes	65 ml	19.5 grams
HYDROCORTISONE (IV/IO/IM) 100 milligrams in 1 ml	100 milligrams	NONE	N/A	1 ml	100 milligrams
HYDROCORTISONE (IV/IO/IM) 100 milligrams in 2 ml	100 milligrams	NONE	N/A	2 ml	100 milligrams
IBUPROFEN (Oral) 100 milligrams in 5 ml	300 milligrams	300 milligrams	8 hours	15 ml	900 milligrams
IPRATROPIUM (Neb) 250 micrograms in 1 ml	250 micrograms	NONE	N/A	1 ml	250 micrograms
IPRATROPIUM (Neb) 500 micrograms in 2 ml	250 micrograms	NONE	N/A	1 ml	250 micrograms
PATIENT'S OWN MIDAZOLAM* (Buccal) 10 milligrams in 1 ml	10 milligrams	NONE	N/A	1 ml	10 milligrams
MORPHINE (IV/IO) 10 milligrams in 10 ml	3 milligrams	3 milligrams	5 minutes	3 ml	6 milligrams
MORPHINE (Oral) 10 milligrams in 5 ml	6 milligrams	NONE	N/A	3 ml	6 milligrams

*Give the dose as prescribed in the child's individualised treatment plan (the dosages described above reflect the recommended dosages for a child of this age).

Drug Therapy

DRUG	INITIAL DOSE	REPEAT DOSE	DOSE INTERVAL	VOLUME	MAXIMUM DOSE
NALOXONE (IV/IO) NB cautions 400 micrograms in 1 ml	320 micrograms	320 micrograms	3 minutes	0.8 ml	3520 micrograms
NALOXONE – INITIAL DOSE (IM) 400 micrograms in 1 ml	320 micrograms	See below	3 minutes	0.8 ml	See below
NALOXONE – REPEAT DOSE (IM) 400 micrograms in 1 ml	–	400 micrograms	–	1 ml	720 micrograms
ONDANSETRON (IV/IO/IM) 2 milligrams in 1 ml	3 milligrams	NONE	N/A	1.5 ml	3 milligrams
PARACETAMOL (Oral) 250 milligrams in 5 ml – six plus suspension	500 milligrams	500 milligrams	4 – 6 hours	10 ml	2 grams in 24 hours
PARACETAMOL (IV/IO) 10 milligrams in 1 ml	500 milligrams	500 milligrams	4 – 6 hours	50 ml	2 grams in 24 hours
SALBUTAMOL (Neb) 2.5 milligrams in 2.5 ml	5 milligrams	5 milligrams	5 minutes	5 ml	No limit
SALBUTAMOL (Neb) 5 milligrams in 2.5 ml	5 milligrams	5 milligrams	5 minutes	2.5 ml	No limit
TRANEXAMIC ACID (IV) 100 mg/ml	500 mg	NONE	N/A	5 ml	500 mg

This page left intentionally blank for your notes

Page for Age

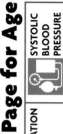

11 YEARS

Vital Signs

	GUIDE WEIGHT	HEART RATE	RESPIRATION RATE	SYSTOLIC BLOOD PRESSURE
	35 kg	80–120	20–25	90–110

Airway Size by Type

OROPHARYNGEAL AIRWAY	LARYNGEAL MASK	I-GEL AIRWAY	ENDOTRACHEAL TUBE
2 OR 3	3	2.5 OR 3	Diameter: **7 mm**; Length: **18 cm**

Defibrillation – Cardiac Arrest

MANUAL	AUTOMATED EXTERNAL DEFIBRILLATOR
140 Joules	A standard AED can be used (without the need for attenuation pads).

Intravascular Fluid

FLUID	INITIAL DOSE	REPEAT DOSE	DOSE INTERVAL	VOLUME	MAXIMUM DOSE
Sodium chloride (5 ml/kg) (IV/IO) 0.9%	175 ml	175 ml	PRN	175 ml	1000 ml
Sodium chloride (10 ml/kg) (IV/IO) 0.9%	350 ml	350 ml	PRN	350 ml	1000 ml
Sodium chloride (20 ml/kg) (IV/IO) 0.9%	500 ml	500 ml	PRN	500 ml	1000 ml

11 YEARS Page for Age

DRUG	INITIAL DOSE	REPEAT DOSE	DOSE INTERVAL	VOLUME	MAXIMUM DOSE
ADRENALINE (IV/IO) 1 milligram in 10 ml (1:10,000)	350 micrograms	350 micrograms	3–5 mins	3.5 ml	No limit
AMIODARONE (IV/IO) 300 milligrams in 10 ml	180 milligrams (after 3rd shock)	180 milligrams	After 5th shock	6 ml	360 milligrams
ATROPINE* (IV/IO) 100 micrograms in 1 ml	500 micrograms	NONE	N/A	5 ml	500 micrograms
ATROPINE* (IV/IO) 200 micrograms in 1 ml	500 micrograms	NONE	N/A	2.5 ml	500 micrograms
ATROPINE* (IV/IO) 300 micrograms in 1 ml	500 micrograms	NONE	N/A	1.7 ml	500 micrograms
ATROPINE* (IV/IO) 600 micrograms in 1 ml	500 micrograms	NONE	N/A	0.8 ml	500 micrograms

***BRADYCARDIA** in children is most commonly caused by **HYPOXIA**, requiring immediate **ABC** care, **NOT** drug therapy; therefore **ONLY** administer atropine in cases of bradycardia caused by vagal stimulation (e.g. suction).

Drug Therapy

DRUG	INITIAL DOSE	REPEAT DOSE	DOSE INTERVAL	VOLUME	MAXIMUM DOSE
ADRENALINE (IM) anaphylaxis/asthma 1 milligram in 1 ml (1:1,000)	300 micrograms	300 micrograms	5 minutes	0.3 ml	No limit
BENZYLPENICILLIN (IV/IO) 600 milligrams in 9.6 ml	1.2 grams	NONE	N/A	20 ml	1.2 grams
BENZYLPENICILLIN (IM) 600 milligrams in 1.6 ml	1.2 grams	NONE	N/A	4 ml	1.2 grams
CHLORPHENAMINE (Oral) Various	2 milligrams	NONE	N/A	N/A	2 milligrams
CHLORPHENAMINE (IV/IO/IM) 10 milligrams in 1 ml	5–10 milligrams	NONE	N/A	0.5 – 1 ml	5 – 10 milligrams
DEXAMETHASONE – croup (Oral)	N/A	N/A	N/A	N/A	N/A
DIAZEPAM (IV/IO) 10 milligrams in 2 ml	10 milligrams	NONE	N/A	2 ml	10 milligrams
DIAZEPAM (PR) 5 milligrams in 2.5 ml or 10 milligrams in 2.5 ml	5 or 10 milligrams	NONE	N/A	1 × 5 milligram tube or 1 × 10 milligram tube	5 or 10 milligrams
GLUCAGON (IM) 1 milligram per vial	1 milligram	NONE	N/A	1 vial	1 milligram

Drug Therapy

DRUG	INITIAL DOSE	REPEAT DOSE	DOSE INTERVAL	VOLUME	MAXIMUM DOSE
GLUCOSE 10% (IV/IO) 50 grams in 500 ml	7 grams	7 grams	5 minutes	70 ml	21 grams
HYDROCORTISONE (IV/IO/IM) 100 milligrams in 1 ml	100 milligrams	NONE	N/A	1 ml	100 milligrams
HYDROCORTISONE (IV/IO/IM) 100 milligrams in 2 ml	100 milligrams	NONE	N/A	2 ml	100 milligrams
IBUPROFEN (Oral) 100 milligrams in 5 ml	300 milligrams	300 milligrams	8 hours	15 ml	900 milligrams
IPRATROPIUM (Neb) 250 micrograms in 1 ml	250 micrograms	NONE	N/A	1 ml	250 micrograms
IPRATROPIUM (Neb) 500 micrograms in 2 ml	250 micrograms	NONE	N/A	1 ml	250 micrograms
PATIENT'S OWN MIDAZOLAM* (Buccal)	10 milligrams	NONE	N/A	1 ml	10 milligrams
MORPHINE (IV/IO) 10 milligrams in 10 ml	3.5 milligrams	3.5 milligrams	5 minutes	3.5 ml	7 milligrams
MORPHINE (Oral) 10 milligrams in 5 ml	7 milligrams	NONE	N/A	3.5 ml	7 milligrams

*Give the dose as prescribed in the child's individualised treatment plan (the dosages described above reflect the recommended dosages for a child of this age).

DRUG	INITIAL DOSE	REPEAT DOSE	DOSE INTERVAL	VOLUME	MAXIMUM DOSE
NALOXONE (IV/IO) NB cautions 400 micrograms in 1 ml	350 micrograms	350 micrograms	3 minutes	0.9 ml	3850 micrograms
NALOXONE – INITIAL DOSE (IM) 400 micrograms in 1 ml	350 micrograms	See below	3 minutes	0.9 ml	See below
NALOXONE – REPEAT DOSE (IM) 400 micrograms in 1 ml	–	400 micrograms	–	1 ml	750 micrograms
ONDANSETRON (IV/IO/IM) 2 milligrams in 1 ml	3 milligrams	NONE	N/A	1.5 ml	3 milligrams
PARACETAMOL (Oral) 250 milligrams in 5 ml – six plus suspension	500 milligrams	500 milligrams	4 – 6 hours	10 ml	2 grams in 24 hours
PARACETAMOL (IV/IO) 10 milligrams in 1 ml	500 milligrams	500 milligrams	4 – 6 hours	50 ml	2 grams in 24 hours
SALBUTAMOL (Neb) 2.5 milligrams in 2.5 ml	5 milligrams	5 milligrams	5 minutes	5 ml	No limit
SALBUTAMOL (Neb) 5 milligrams in 2.5 ml	5 milligrams	5 milligrams	5 minutes	2.5 ml	No limit
TRANEXAMIC ACID (IV) 100 mg/ml	500 mg	NONE	N/A	5 ml	500 mg

Notes

Notes